Communicating
PLANTS

"*Communicating with Plants* is Jen's love letter to both people and plants. She artfully and heartfully shares her experience and perspective as she answers one of the questions I am asked most frequently, 'How do I listen to a plant?' She demystifies the process and teaches the simplicity and naturalness of our innate ability to communicate and commune with these elders, teachers, and healers who love us and have so much to offer when we take the time to listen. As Jen shares with her readers, our relationships with the plants restore us to ourselves, and this benefits us, them, and all beings on our beautiful Earth. I am grateful that Jen Frey wrote this book; it also provides specific plant wisdom that can help readers on their journey of remembering themselves as part of Nature."

ROBIN ROSE BENNETT, HERBALIST AND
AUTHOR OF *THE GIFT OF HEALING HERBS*

"Jen Frey is a committed long-term ally of the plant world. Her sensitivity and direct knowledge of the plants inspire. Her account of interspecies communication vibrates with authenticity and love. As a sensitive being in a vital world, Jen leads us to a world of wonderment."

WILLIAM MORRIS, PH.D., DAOM, HERBALIST AND AUTHOR OF
TRANSFORMATION: TREATING TRAUMA WITH ACUPUNCTURE AND HERBS

"In her generous new book *Communicating with Plants,* Jen Frey affirms that the world of plants can be not only food and medicine for humanity but also companions, guardians, and teachers as well. Taking plants as her muse, Jen proceeds to teach us not only about the healing properties of these more-than-human neighbors but also through the lens of the plant she touches on some of life's most important lessons: to live with an open heart, to be aware of subtle energies, to honor and work with dreams, to befriend our own wildness, and much more. For anyone who loves the green Earth and wants to deepen into relationship with plants, Jen's book will be a bountiful exploration."

SHARIFA OPPENHEIMER, AUTHOR OF
A LITANY OF WILD GRACES: MEDITATIONS ON SACRED ECOLOGY

"A wonderful book has come our way. Jen Frey's *Communicating with Plants* is an inspiration. When a book is written with as much intelligence and deep insight as this one, the result is a special treat. Congratulations, this is a book to take people into the Light. Oh, and incidentally . . . I also am very connected with Mulberry!"

MICHAEL J. ROADS, AUTHOR OF
TALKING WITH NATURE AND *JOURNEY INTO NATURE*

"Jen has given us a tremendous gift being the plant's pencil. This intimate and profound guide for entering into relationship with our kin—the plants—will help anyone move into a deeper relationship, wherever they are in their plant journey. Reading this book will change you. Reading this book may save you."

TAMMI SWEET, AUTHOR OF
THE WHOLISTIC HEALING GUIDE TO CANNABIS
AND CODIRECTOR OF THE HEARTSTONE
CENTER FOR EARTH ESSENTIALS

"Some writers have the gift of storytelling—their words are conversational, intimate, and captivating. I felt my fairy godmother had me in her lap, winding the path of wisdom transformed into sensations, opening my eyes, the windows of my soul, to the deeply felt world of plants. Within this book you will read passages potent with analogies of truth. At last, solutions and hope in harmony with our ancestors."

MARGI FLINT, AUTHOR OF *THE PRACTICING HERBALIST*

"Brilliantly written from the heart, this book gives readers a series of exercises that open us to understanding what the plants want us to know. The author takes a subject that is often dismissed and makes it accessible and solid. Jen Frey let the plants speak through her, and now we only need to pay attention."

TINA SAMS, AUTHOR OF *THE BIG BOOK OF HERBAL MEDICINE*

"There are special people sensitive enough to hear the conversations happening all around us between our green kin. The plants choose these folk to speak for them—to translate their meanings and intentions into words. Jen Frey is one of these people. She straddles both worlds and generously shares her ways of making those connections. A heartwarming book."

MARY REYNOLDS, FOUNDER OF THE GLOBAL MOVEMENT
WE ARE THE ARK AND AUTHOR OF *THE GARDEN AWAKENING*

Communicating with PLANTS

Heart-Based Practices for Connecting with Plant Spirits

Jen Frey

Illustrated by Lillian Edwards

Bear & Company
Rochester, Vermont

Bear & Company
One Park Street
Rochester, Vermont 05767
www.BearandCompanyBooks.com

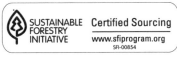

Text stock is SFI certified

Bear & Company is a division of Inner Traditions International

Cataloging-in-Publication Data for this title is available from the Library of Congress

ISBN 978-1-59143-459-7 (print)
ISBN 978-1-59143-460-3 (ebook)

Printed and bound in the United States by Lake Book Manufacturing, LLC
The text stock is SFI certified. The Sustainable Forestry Initiative® program
promotes sustainable forest management.

10 9 8 7 6 5 4 3 2 1

Text design by Virginia Scott Bowman and layout by Priscilla Harris Baker
This book was typeset in Garamond Premier Pro with Angie Sans, Gill Sans, Late
Fall, and Matrix II
Black and white illustrations by Lillian Edwards

To send correspondence to the author of this book, mail a first-class letter to the
author c/o Inner Traditions • Bear & Company, One Park Street, Rochester, VT
05767, and we will forward the communication, or contact the author directly at
www.brigidsway.com.

*For Alex
and future generations*

❧ Contents ☙

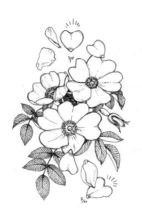

❧ The Legacy ❧ of Plant Spirits

"*I* owe my life to Plants" is a profound way to begin this testament to the green beings. Jen Frey, in her book *Communicating with Plants,* is not only being literal when she makes this declaration but is also opening a wide-angle lens on the numinous nature of plants and trees. Our symbiotic relationship with plants is undeniable on all levels, physically, emotionally, mentally, and spiritually.

Because plants are uniquely photosynthetic they provide us with all our basic physical needs. Through photosynthesis they capture sunlight and use this energy to extract carbon dioxide (which we exhale) from the atmosphere then combine it with water to form sugars that make leaves, stalks, roots, seeds, and flowers, which contain starch, fat, and protein. The by-product of this process is oxygen. Plants are the *only* source of oxygen. All of our breath comes from plants, all of our tissue comes from plants, all of our food comes from plants. We are completely dependent on plants for our basic physical needs.

On an emotional level our symbiosis can be understood through biophilia, otherwise known as the love of nature. Biophilia comes from both our similarity to plants and our symbiosis with nature and our long and close association with nature and plants throughout the emergence of our human species. There is thought to be an inherited, genetic need to be in close proximity to that which gives you your life—nature and plants. Through this close association a type of bond occurs that is necessary for healthy gaiacology (relationship with a living Earth). Deep healing can take place by being with what you love, what nurtures you and what gives you your very life. We are touched by our genetically inherited love for green beings and we are healed by their love for us.

On a mental level because our ancient plant ancestors were able to communicate and organize themselves to grow, reproduce, inherit, and mutate (adapt) they developed self-awareness, which lies at the heart of the origins of consciousness. Many biologists now believe that the rise in higher types of psychological behavior culminating in mind is a result of plants initiating self-awareness over 2 billion years ago. They developed very sophisticated and complex communication abilities that include being able to compute and make decisions about complex aspects of their environment; intricate signaling systems to alert neighbors; foraging and competing for resources; and, through large protein molecules, the ability to store large amounts of information allowing for an enormous capacity for complexity in communication and retention of data, and remembering all of this to set future intentions of intelligent choice. They can learn, remember, and decide without a so-called brain—and this all began prior to human evolution.

Spirit, the vital principle, held to give life, as a hologram helps us understand that we are a part of that which is greater than ourselves and that we carry the whole of that greatness within us. When we look at the big picture, we see that plants have always preceded their animal counterparts in evolution. Our evolution is now one of raising our consciousness on a spiritual level so that we feed life instead of destroying it. Plants continue to set the precedent by guiding us in our spiritual evolution. In their own evolution they are stepping up to become our Elders and have taken on the role of initiating us into becoming truly human, living within our true essential nature, walking the path we came for in order to take up our rightful place as a part of nature. Nature is the ultimate in vital force, with plants being the aspect of nature we are most related to so that via the plants we have easy access to spirit. Our very life-giving vitality—spirit—comes directly from the plants.

In *Communicating with Plants,* Jen weaves this deep symbiotic relationship with plants and trees throughout her stories. Her stories are contemporary and yet carry the bio-intelligence of the ages where a living conversation with the natural world both seen and unseen comes alive with the potent awareness that this is our birthright. As we marinate in Jen's wisdom words we realize that we actually *do* know how to communicate with the natural world, especially our closest of kin, the plants and trees. When we settle into the common union that communication brings we begin to remember who we truly are. We remember the legacy of the plants and how crucially important it is to not only remember this legacy but to continue to pass it on.

This is one of the reasons we write books, tell our stories, and strive to know the plants and their magnanimous spirits at a deep level—so the legacy of the plants can be carried on. Jen has become a torch bearer for this legacy by honoring not only her human plant-loving ancestors but also the plants themselves as our ancestors. These green being ancestors were the first living organisms on this planet so they carry the long view with the stories of the ages imbedded in their multidimensional essence. Jen has listened with "big ears" to her kin and is exalting their legacy through her rich and insightful stories while illuminating some of their forgotten gifts.

When I first met Jen it felt like I had known her for lifetimes. We immediately recognized each other as Earth sisters who deeply love the natural world. She became my apprentice and was a quick study and so, before long, she became one of my teacher assistants, helping me with apprentice programs, classes, and online courses. She has gone on to teach her own apprentice programs, bringing the teachings of Plant Spirit Healing to a wide audience. It is not surprising that now she is helping to bring Plant Spirits into "the commons" where these sentient beings take up their place within consensus reality and we all agree they are indeed our wise Elders who are guiding us in our consciousness-raising evolution.

Written in easy to understand terms, *Communicating with Plants* speaks to the novice and yet the seasoned plant lover will be moved by Jen's deep insights and profound understanding. As we delve into this potent book we begin to wake up from our amnesia and remember not only who we are, but also who the plants are to us. In Jen's words, "As we connect with the Plants, they help us to remember our Sacred role as part of Nature, which ultimately reminds us of who we are. Our connection helps us to align with our Soul's path, re-membering our wholeness. We have been wandering for so long that sometimes we forget that we are lost. Still the Plants continue to gently call us back to ourselves, to our Sacred family. They believe in our ability to return to the Garden and, like any fabulous relative, they will continue to remind us of our Truth, until we can remember for ourselves."

Plants have a natural affinity with the heart. Since the heart is the primary organ of perception it receives all the touches from the plants. Jen brings heart to her work with the plants but not in a maudlin or trivial way. Jen's heart-centered approach to plant communication is like a healing balm on the fractures caused by the crushing impact of modern-day life. When we lead with our heart we realize we are actually quite resilient and don't need to fall prey to heartbreaking realities. The brilliance of our heart saves us every time. As Jen writes, "When we communicate with Plants, we want to be in our Heart space, accessing our Heart's intelligence. . . . This intelligence is intuitive, creative, cooperative, solution oriented, perceptive, imaginative, and focuses on the gift." Is it possible that plants can teach us how to live with heart intelligence in *all* of our communications? Can you imagine what our world would be like if we engaged with heart intelligence every day?

We are so fortunate to have allies like the plants who "have our backs" and to have someone like Jen Frey who is courageous enough to be the champion for these life-saving green beings. As Jen guides us to take our already existing relationship with the plants and trees to the next level of partnership we realize how profound this connection actually is. We would not have our life if not for this nature alliance. As we learn the language of plants and communication becomes intrinsic we delight in a partnership so deep that the green beings become our beloveds. Together we can move into a co-creative partnership where we combine our gifts for all of life to thrive.

Thank you, Jen, for this blessing of a book that helps us find our way back home to the plants and trees who are our kin, our friends, our beloveds, our teachers, our partners in life.

PAM MONTGOMERY, AUTHOR OF *PLANT SPIRIT HEALING:*
A GUIDE TO WORKING WITH PLANT CONSCIOUSNESS
DANBY, VERMONT
MARCH 2022

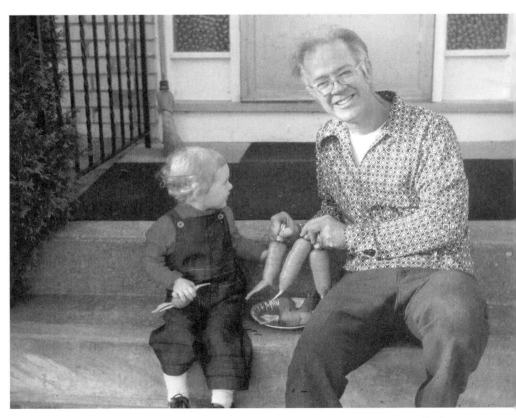

Author as a toddler, looking adoringly at her maternal grandfather and his prized Carrots.

❧ An Invitation ❧
into the Plant World

I owe my life to Plants.

This is a simple statement and yet, can you feel the power in it? The truth is that while Plants have been the cornerstone of my life since I was quite young, we all owe our lives to Plants. Plants make this amazing, wonderful, fantastic planet livable. Among many gifts, they provide the oxygen that we need to breathe. Have you ever pondered this miracle? Have you ever breathed with a Plant or truly recognized the connection between Plants and your life?

When I do this, the word that comes to my mind is Love.

Some of my more scientifically inclined friends and colleagues would caution me against this or at the very least would start to squirm in their seats at the idea. They would say that we humans have a tendency towards anthropomorphism, assigning emotions and relationships to other species that do not exist other than through our human lens.

After spending many years communicating with Plants and having my life guided by them, I think Love is an accurate word.

I know that I am not alone. Talk with any true Plant lover about Plants and you will start to see the twinkle in their eye. I love Plant people. We come in many shapes, sizes, colors, and economic levels. We have various religious backgrounds and political beliefs. We can have greatly differing opinions on the best way to interact with Plants or grow them. However, all the differences and disagreements are quickly forgotten when we begin to talk about a well-loved Plant. In that moment, when the guard goes down and the Heart opens, we understand that this other person has experienced the magic of Plants. Once this magic is experienced, our lives are forever changed.

Numerous people have shared their stories with me about their childhood relationships with Plants and Nature. They were aware of magical worlds and knew a different language. Then they went to school or their families discovered their relationships, and they gave up their connections to fit into the societal norms and expectations. As they tell me their stories, their faces reveal a deep heartbrokenness, for they long to have that connection again. I'll share with you what I tell them: you have not lost anything. The connection remains, the path is there, and, though it may be a little grown over, you can rediscover it more easily than you think. The Plants are waiting for you. I have yet to meet someone who was not able to return to the magical world of Plants. It is never too late, nor is the path ever completely lost.

As for myself and my own path, I have had a lifelong love affair with Plants. Really, I don't know if I had a choice. Both of my grandfathers loved gardening and Plants. In their unique ways, they introduced me to the magic of Plants. From a young age, Plants were a solace, and as I got older, they became my teachers, my Guides, my medicine, and my friends. After all these years with them, I know that I am barely scratching the surface of their wisdom, gifts, and our relationship. Every day that I am able to spend time with them is a gift that I cherish. They have brought me back from the deepest depths of pain, lovingly chastised me when I was not listening, and have brought me great joy and pleasure. No matter how much I messed up or would try to ignore them, the Plants continued to show up, again and again.

My apprenticeship with the Plants became serious when I purchased my dream property in 2003. It took almost a year before my family could live there, but I quickly planted a garden and started to observe the wild Plants. In the spring and summer of 2005, I spent my mornings harvesting berries. While harvesting, information would come to me, problems that I had been stewing over suddenly seemed clear, and I found a deep calm. The idea that I should write a book about Plants came to me, but in my humility I quickly discounted it—I was in my twenties and didn't think I had anything to share about Plants; there were people who were much wiser and had more life experience than me and they were the ones who should be writing.

At this time, I also did not believe that I could communicate with Plants. To be clear, I did believe, whole-heartedly, that some people were capable of Plant communication, but that I simply was not one of them. Little did I know that the solutions to my problems, the idea to write a book—all of the messages that I had been receiving—were the Plants communicating with me. Several years ago, I realized that my "humility" was actually arrogance, because it wasn't me who was supposed to write; the Plants were asking to write the book through me.

Now I am endeavoring to be the Plants' pencil. Since the early berry picking days, I have become a voice for the Plants and have taught many people how to communicate with them. I believe that Plant communication is, as Pam Montgomery says, our birthright. *Everyone* has the innate ability to communicate with Plants.

If you are reading this and thinking, "This is bizarre!" that's fine. You are not the first person to think that. I invite you to put your disbelief aside and simply wonder, "What if?—what if Plants could communicate with us?" Or perhaps you will read my stories as fairy tales; you do not need to believe that what I write is true.

If you are reading this and thinking, "That's cool, but I'm sure I am not able to do this," or wish that you had this skill, I assure you, you can and you do. The Plants communicate with us all the time. The difference between me today and me in 2005 is that I am now able to recognize the ways that the Plants are communicating. If you think that you are not one of the "special" people who can communicate with Plants, I ask you to please put that thought aside. I have taught Plant communication in various forms for around fifteen years to people of all ages and I've never had someone who did not receive information from a Plant. There are those who want to make this out to be a complicated process and it just isn't. Again, communicating with Plants (really all of Nature) is your birthright. What I tell my students is that my job is to help them overcome the culturalization that tells them they are unable to communicate with Plants and help them remember this innate skill. Once we get rid of these blockages, the rest is easy.

For those of you who have already experienced the wonders of the Plant world, may my words be the magic dust that brings your own adventures to life and gives encouragement to delve deeper.

You see, we are a bunch of amnesiacs. This is no fault of our own. It is our nature. By the time we take our first breath on this Earth, we have already forgotten much of the wisdom of the universe. As we grow, the amnesia takes over like a giant eraser until we no longer know who we are or why we are here. Unfortunately, most of our Ancestors were also amnesiacs, so for generations we have been losing more and more Sacred knowledge, without even realizing it. Then, of course, there are those of us whose Ancestors had their wisdom stolen, beaten, and murdered out of them, usually in the name of money, religion, or progress.

I share this statement of our amnesia as a message of hope. For once we realize what we are experiencing, we can then choose a different way and remember. We can also stop the blame or self-sabotage, understanding that this is simply who we are and focusing our energy toward our remembering. We do not get angry with a baby because they don't know how to talk or walk. We support and celebrate their learning and growing. We should extend this grace to ourselves.

Fortunately, there are humans (and cultures) who have managed to keep the threads of Sacred knowledge alive. We need to honor them and protect them, which means protecting their Lands, their languages, and their traditions. If we are invited, we can also learn from them. This remembering is too much for any one person or group of people to do—it is a collective endeavor.

Many of the younger generations are being born with more Sacred memory. We need to protect them and raise them with Love and reverence in a way that keeps their Souls intact and honors their Sacred roles as catalysts and awakeners. Sadly, many of them are given labels and medicated to try to make them conform to our amnesiac ways, rather than having their gifts recognized and heeded. We want to listen to these wise young ones and also do our own work. It is not fair to hand the problems of the world to the younger generation, hoping that they will "fix" them. We have an active role in the remembering.

We can learn from the same Source who helped our Ancestors and the Wise Ones alive today: the Earth herself, including Plants, rocks, waters, animals. . . . They are able to help us to heal, to learn, to grow, and to remember who we are, why we are here, and how we can live in harmony with all Beings. With their help, we re-member the future.

One word of caution: our amnesia makes us hungry. We know that something is missing (often on an unconscious level). We try to fill this void through consumption, of anything and everything. This is quite obvious when we look at our relationship with Earth—clear cutting old growth Forests and the Amazon Rainforest; mining for gems, minerals, and coal; fracking and sucking out the last drops of petroleum; the accumulation of islands of plastic floating in the ocean; and so on. It's also evident in the enormous role addiction plays in our lives, including television, shopping, food, alcohol, drugs, pornography, sugar, caffeine, and sex.

A less obvious form is our consumption of ideas, information, and experiences, which can sometimes take the form of appropriation. Sometimes we witness or we hear about someone who has a profound relationship with Nature, and our hunger pulls us to them like vultures to a freshly killed deer; we want to consume them and their wisdom hoping that this will fill the void and that we can remember our relationship with Spirit through them. But it doesn't work. It feels as if our hunger is satiated for a little while, but we then follow the scent to the next Wise One or ceremony. Ultimately, we remain hungry.

We cannot consume our way to Spirit nor to our remembering. These actions only deepen our amnesia. I have witnessed this attempt at filling up quite often and have been both the consumer and the consumed. I can tell you that it does not feel good, that no one is served by this endless consuming. If you are finding yourself looking for the next "fix," the next ceremony, the next medicine person, the next experience that will help you to awaken, I invite you to pause, slow down, and recognize the amnesia. We must do our own personal work, healing our traumas and listening to our Soul.

Mostly, I have been talking about the interactions of people; however, the same is absolutely true when we interact with Earth. The Plants are overwhelmingly generous Beings. We can get caught up in having experiences with or knowing a large number of Plants, or focusing on having incredibly intense interactions with Plants, which feeds the amnesia.

Receiving wisdom or a profound healing or experiencing a Sacred ceremony is an enormous gift. With that gift comes responsibility. It is an opportunity to remember your wholeness and your own innate relationship with Spirit, which is how we truly satiate the hunger. Generally, we need time to allow this gift to infuse into ourselves, to truly digest and understand it. Then we can discover what the gift is requiring of us. What we do with the gift, how we uphold our responsibility, is essential. Do we share this with others? Do we need to make a shift in our own life? The re-membering occurs through our response.

This does not mean that we should never aim to learn from someone else. We simply need to be mindful of why we are seeking. Is this a Heart calling or are we ego driven? Is our consumption keeping us from listening to or healing a wound, pain, or trauma? As I said, I have been a consumer, and perhaps I will be again in the future. There is no shame in this. It is simply a sign that I am experiencing amnesia and my Soul is not being fed.

When we are in right relationship with Plants and Earth, we naturally flow out of the consumer mind frame. We move into intimacy. We want to honor them and be of service to them. The Plants help us to remember our Sacred role as *part* of Nature, clearing away the amnesia.

Each of us engaged in this work adds a few threads to our collective awakening. Sometimes our threads are similar to others and sometimes our pieces inspire someone else or help them to understand their experiences. We need as many people as possible to listen, learn, heal, and remember so that we can weave our future together.

I offer you this book as part of the remembering.

The Plants are offering us guidance to help us live and thrive during this unique time on Earth and to help us to create a more beautiful and healthier world. The Plants included in this book are here because they asked to be and because they have been important in my life. There are many others who have touched my life in extraordinary ways. There may be other Plants who are more important to you. While we are all connected, we are all different. This is part of what makes life enjoyable. Trust who shows up for you and the wisdom they share that is specific for you.

As humans we like to categorize everything into hierarchical groups, which helps us to understand this expansive world. However, Nature does not work that way. While the Plants included here are most definitely special, they are no more or less special than any other Plant. Each has a unique role for our planet, for humanity, and for our evolution.

I share examples of how the Plants' messages have manifested in my life as well as my clients' and students' lives. This is to help give more context and understanding to the lessons from the Plants. These are only examples; there are many different ways in which you can incorporate the Plants' guidance into your life. I encourage you to allow these messages to take the form that you need most; in other words, make them your own.

This book also acts as your personal Plant Communication Guide; use it in conjunction with your own wisdom. Ideally, you will work with one Plant as you go through this guide. At the end of each chapter, you will find an exercise to help you connect and communicate with your Plant ally. Each exercise provides another piece of the puzzle for understanding and communicating with your Plant. You may find that you resonate well with some of the exercises while others are a struggle. This is fine. There is no one way to communicate with Plants; we all have our own unique journey. However, I do encourage you to at least attempt them, as you may find a new way of relating or learn something about yourself in the process. You can move at your own pace through the exercises; I encourage you to take your time. This process is about moving into intimacy with a Plant and intimacy requires an investment of energy, including time. The organization of the exercises is similar to how I teach them in my classes; they often build on one another. It is imperative that you are in Heart coherence when connecting with your Plant; therefore, please begin with the first two exercises, "Accessing Your Heart Space" and "The First Meeting." However, this is your experience, so after these first two exercises, feel free to shift the order to what works best for you.

I have witnessed that some people need more assistance than others in the beginning. Some very fortunate people never forgot how to communicate with other species. Others simply need permission and perhaps a few tricks to remember. Some can attend one of my introductory classes, where we do not practice any of the exercises, and are able to go home and open themselves to a whole new world. Still others need more guidance, which is mostly assurance that they are capable and perhaps need help translating their experiences. Therefore, if you try my suggestions and feel like you aren't connecting or receiving anything, I encourage you to participate in a class or have someone mentor you in person.

Plants come into our lives in amazing ways and each has much to offer us. The best herb books have a chapter written about each Plant; in reality, however, each Plant could have their own encyclopedia if we are willing to continue to listen and see them with new eyes. Plants meet us where we are. Our Plant ally will reveal new gifts and understandings as we heal, evolve, and move through changing life circumstances. Therefore, we could have a group of people communicating with the same Plant and each person could receive different messages. This wouldn't mean that people are not communicating "correctly" or that those messages are inaccurate. Simply, the Plant is offering to each individual the information that they need most at that time.

The most important thing is to have fun and enjoy the gifts the Plants have to offer you.

I focus on communicating with Plants because I have found them to be the easiest introduction into communicating with Nature. Plants are relatively stationary. They are our Ancestors. They have lived on this planet for much longer than humans and survived several major planetary changes. They are great adaptors and they tend to have a much broader, longer view than humans. They generally enjoy humans. They have an incredibly generous and forgiving nature. Plants know how to live in community and work with other species. They acknowledge their role as guides for humanity. Once you are comfortable communicating with Plants, it becomes easier to communicate with the other Nature Beings (including humans). Of course, there are those who are more attuned to animals or rocks or Elemental Beings. If this is you, that's wonderful! Please continue communicating in the manner that feels best for you. You can use this book to broaden your communication abilities to Plants or simply digest the messages that the Plants want to share.

As we connect with the Plants, they help us to remember our Sacred role as part of Nature, which ultimately reminds us of who we are. Our connection helps us to align with our Soul's path, re-membering our wholeness. We have been wandering for so long that sometimes we forget that we are lost. Still the Plants continue to gently call us back to ourselves, to our Sacred family. They believe in our ability to return to the Garden and, like any fabulous relative, they will continue to remind us of our Truth, until we can remember for ourselves.

And now, I invite you to breathe deeply, taking in this life-giving gift from the Plants.

Come to the Forest

Come to the Forest, my friend
Breathe in the mist
Let your lungs fill with the Green Mystery
Let your cells expand
Let your feet sink into the Humus
Let your roots grow
Feel them mingle with the Mycelium
Let them merge with Tree roots and

Tap into the Ancient Wisdom
Allow your hairs to become antennae,
Sensing the invisible
Your wings begin to sprout
Completing the transformation
As your Heart awakens and
Becomes Wild
Again

A Note on Capitalization, Ki, and Gender

One of my goals in life is to help elevate Plants and other aspects of Nature in our awareness. We have a tendency to think of them and treat them as unintelligent, inanimate objects. This allows us to make decisions without taking their well-being into consideration (such as cutting down a Forest). Therefore, I choose to capitalize their names as if they are human. For the purpose of this book and to create an easier reading experience, I am limiting the capitalization of some aspects of Nature, mostly focusing on those connected to Plants and a few other words that I believe could use more emphasis and awareness in our culture, such as Heart, Love, and Soul.

Language is an integral part of how we experience the world. The words we speak, the sounds we make, literally shape us. Their vibrations resonate both internally and externally also affecting the world around us. Language is also limiting; it is difficult to distill large experiences felt on many levels into words. As society evolves, so does our language. Words go out of fashion or are deemed too harmful. We create new words to better explain our current world. Adjusting our language helps us to discern what we value and, ultimately, helps us to create the world.

The language we use affects our relationships. Since Plants, animals, and the other Beings are alive, I choose (as best as I can) to use animistic language. Therefore, I refer to them as "ki" instead of "it." To the best of my knowledge, this word was first suggested as an animistic, genderless pronoun by Robin Wall Kimmerer.[1] After years of using this pronoun, I can notice an effect on how I view and think about Nature. I invite you to experiment with using the word *ki*. In my daily life, I sometimes refer to Plants as they, she, or he—though, since gender is a human construct, Plants are neither male nor female. In fact, many Plants fluidly shift between what we consider to be male (pollen-producing) and female (fruit-producing). I admit that sometimes I do refer to Plants as it. Mostly this is for easier comprehension, but sometimes I also slip back into the old pattern of "it."

While we are on the subject of gender, let's talk about humans. Since I was young, gender seemed like a strange concept to me. It seems a shame to try to cram a beautiful rainbow into a binary box. I am glad that we are beginning to shift our understanding around gender. We are multidimensional Beings—why put limitations on us?

Having said that, I am fully aware that our understanding of and language around gender is evolving, sometimes quickly and sometimes painfully slowly. My worldview and language shift as I continue to learn, heal, and move beyond my conditioning. Please know that my intention is to be inclusive and honoring of all Beings and their magnificent expressions. In this book, I rarely refer to men and women, mostly because, again, this is not a concept that the Plants utilize. They relate to the wholeness of you. They see your Soul, which is genderless. You, Dear Reader, know yourself better than I. Please feel free to put yourself in whichever description feels most appropriate to you, including none of them.

Ultimately, this book is meant as an offering of Love: an offering of Love from the Plants to you, an offering of Love from me to you, and an offering of Love from me to the Plants. My hope is that you feel this and know that you are Love(d).

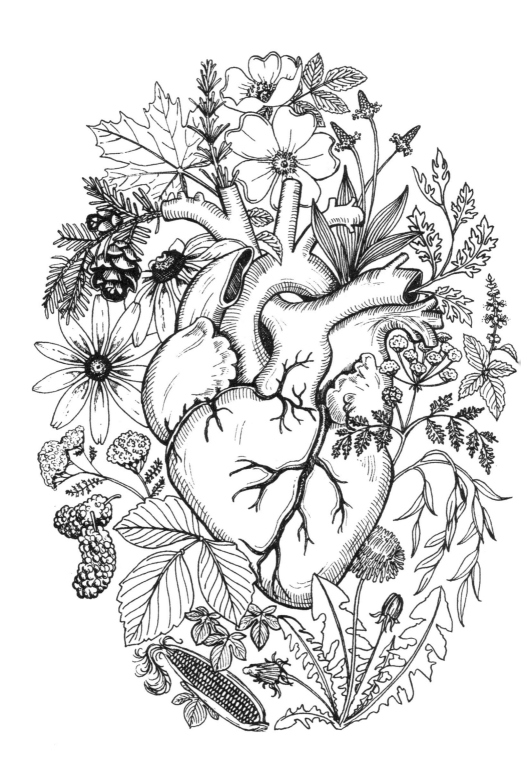

1

❧ Plant Communication ❧

We are living during a time of great opportunity and change. If we want to thrive, if we want to succeed, we need to learn how to live in co-creative partnership with Nature. Plants can show us how to do this and, more importantly, they want to help us do this. If I had my way, Plant communication would be taught in school along with reading and writing. Our future depends on our ability to communicate with other species. Plants can help us to discover solutions to any problem or question, including big collective issues such as climate change, social injustice, energy alternatives, poverty, agriculture, housing, diseases, and anything else that keeps us from thriving. When communicating with Plants, we each bring our own experiences and skills into the relationship, enabling us to ask a variety of questions and discover the possibilities within our areas of expertise. Plants meet us where we are, sharing the wisdom and gifts that we need the most at that time. Therefore, it is imperative to our shared future that everyone remembers how to communicate with Plants. Together we weave the wisdom we receive to create the world of our dreams.

There are many wonderful modalities and systems that are designed to help humans live in a way that is less damaging or, ideally, healing to the Earth, such as regenerative agriculture, biodynamics, and permaculture. These are great and offer solutions to many of our problems. However, if we are not communicating with Nature as we go forward with our efforts, then we continue to engage in a human dominant culture (aka "humansplaining"). When we work in alignment with Nature, the work becomes easier and is more effective.

Embracing Our Birthright

Throughout my life I heard stories of people who were able to communicate with Plants. I hoped that one day, if I worked hard, I too would be able to have this amazing skill. I read books by people who wrote about their ability to communicate with the Plant world. At one point, I had a teacher who taught me a long and intricate process; however, try as I might, I didn't really understand it, which only confirmed my belief that this gift was beyond my capability.

Little did I know that no work is required to obtain this skill. We are born with the innate ability to communicate with Plants (and other Beings). In fact, in the simplest terms, with every breath we take, we receive information from the Plants. As is typical for us humans, we tend to make this more difficult than it is.

Here's the important part: Plants want to communicate with us. They love us. They know their part in the great web of Life, and they want to help us remember ours.

How can we be in good relationship with Plants (or Nature) if we do not know how to communicate with them? And what are we missing when we are unable to receive their messages?

I can say for me, I was missing a lot! Since realizing that I am able to communicate with Plants, I have received an enormous amount of Love, understanding, and guidance. The Plants have been my biggest support through some of the toughest times in my life. And they have also helped me to grow. My relationship with them has given me a greater understanding about who I am and how the universe works, and opened me up to an unbelievable amount of pleasure. Before I remembered this skill, I felt lost and uncertain. I still feel uncertain sometimes; however, now I know that I am never alone and I always have access to support and guidance. I know that my experience is not unique. Time and again, my students and clients have told me that learning how to communicate with Plants has changed their lives. Remembering this skill has brought back aspects of themselves that they thought had disappeared forever.

I wish that I could truly relay how grateful I am to have this relationship with the Plants. All I can do is to encourage you on this path of connection and trust that you too will discover the magic.

Communication—Communion—Common Union

What is communication? When I teach Plant communication, I write the above words on the board. I received this nugget from Pam Montgomery. This breakdown is a good reminder of what we experience when we communicate or at least what we hope to experience. Perhaps that alone can help us to communicate more effectively.

The root of communication is communion or common union. When we communicate, we move into communion, we connect. While we can receive incredible information from the Plants, I think the most important aspect is this communion—for this is what reminds us of our connection to everything, helps us remember our place in this great web of Life, and adds a layer of beauty and depth to our existence.

Recall a great conversation that you had with another person. How did you feel? Those conversations that uplift us or make us feel seen or connected to another person move us into the place of communion. We sense this even if we do not have words for it. During communion, our Hearts become entrained or synchronized; they move into rhythm together, connecting us, facilitating communication and the sharing of our energies.

Our Hearts are the biggest oscillator of the body. In elementary school, we learned that if you had a room filled with pendulums of different sizes and you started them moving at different speeds, eventually they would begin to move together at the same speed, matching the rhythm of the largest pendulum or oscillator. When our Heart is in coherence, ki helps the other organs of our bodies to be healthier. Our Heart's electromagnetic field can be measured outside of our body;

therefore, our coherent Heart can help another person's Heart become coherent, bringing us into union.

Now let's recall a conversation with someone where you are not understanding one another, perhaps it's an argument or perhaps you both keep saying the same thing and not feeling heard. How does this feel? Do you feel the communion? Of course not. Your Hearts are not entrained, you are not connected, and, therefore, communication is not occurring. However, if you take a moment to pause, breathe, and focus on something that you appreciate about the other person, you may discover that it becomes easier to have the conversation. Looking into each other's eyes, holding hands or touching (even if it's the tips of our shoes), and reminiscing about a fun, shared moment together helps our Hearts to entrain. You may each need to practice active listening and perhaps reflecting. Still, we can see that having a coherent Heart and entraining our Heart with someone else's facilitates communication and connection.

Plants excel at entrainment. If our Heart is coherent, they will tune themselves to us, enabling communication to flow. It is possible to communicate with Plants when our Hearts aren't coherent; however, it is more difficult and we are likely to miss the gifts that they are sharing.

The foundation for good communication is listening. There is a large difference between hearing and listening. When you listen, you assimilate all the cues, you are fully present, not wondering what to say next or, even worse, wondering what you are going to make for dinner. The same is true for Plant communication: the basis is listening. Again, the Plants communicate with us all the time, we just tend to not pay attention.

If we want to be more successful in our communication with Plants, Nature, or really any Being (including humans), it is important to understand the ways in which we receive information. Communication is broader than verbalizing, hearing, reading, or writing words. We receive information in varied ways, including through observation. For instance, we learn more from facial expressions and body language than we do from the words that we hear.

All True Communication Begins in the Heart

We forget this. Our society is based on the outdated paradigm of separation. To support this myth, the Heart, the organ of connection and perception, has been considered frivolous, while the brain is put on a pedestal for its capability of thought and logic. And so we believe that communication occurs via thinking a thought, using the vocal cords to share this thought, and someone hearing this with their ears. Travel to a foreign country or spend time with a young child and you quickly remember the many methods of communicating. A lot can be said by simply looking into a person's eyes.

Our Hearts are our main organ of perception. There are numerous studies that show that our Heart responds before our brain and informs the brain about how to respond. This small, incredibly strong organ that has been abused and chided for centuries is one of our greatest tools.

The Heart has ki's own form of intelligence. This intelligence is intuitive, creative, cooperative, solution oriented, perceptive, imaginative, and focuses on the gift. When we are able to be in our Heart center or experience Heart coherence, our nervous system calms down, cortisol levels drop, DHEA (an anti-aging hormone) increases, our breathing deepens and slows, our body relaxes, our stress lessens, and we move into a receptive state (instead of reactionary). The more we can stay in Heart coherence, the happier we are and the easier it is for us to bond and connect with others, as well as experience bliss.

Life is full of challenges and difficulties. How we respond to these or experience them depends largely on our perspective, which is affected by the state of our Heart. Let's look at an example. If you lost your job, it would be completely understandable to freak out about this. Perhaps your thoughts begin to spiral: "How can I afford my mortgage? Can I even afford rent? If we lose our house, my partner will leave me. Maybe I need to move in with my parents. I will lose my health insurance too, and if I don't have health insurance, I can't pay for my child's medication or their doctor's visits . . ." In a scenario like this, we think about everything that *may* go wrong, often inflating the situation to the worst possible outcome. Or we might direct our concerns outward, blaming others—"I'm suffering because of my boss or a co-worker or something that happened five years ago."

If we can pause, access our Heart intelligence, and look again, we might be able to see the situation differently. Perhaps you realize that you were miserable in this job and had been wanting to make a change for years, but were afraid to do it. Perhaps you got into arguments with your partner at night because you were tired and stressed from work, or never had time to do what you really wanted. Perhaps you were offered a severance package that can buy you some time to start your own company, or perhaps you want to change careers or go back to school.

The facts are the same in both scenarios; the only difference is how we look at them. When we access our Heart intelligence, we see and experience the world in a completely different way. The first response focuses on the problem—I lost my job. The second response focuses on the opportunities offered by the change—I can create a situation where I am happier. The second scenario also demonstrates a greater access to creativity and imagination, allowing you to see a broader perspective and recognize the gift.

When we communicate with Plants, we want to be in our Heart space, accessing our Heart's intelligence. This enables us to more easily receive and recognize the communication that is occurring.

Moving into Heart Coherence

We can access our Heart intelligence when our Hearts are in a coherent state; in other words, when our heart rate variability (variation in time between heartbeats) is coherent and ordered. You can purchase apps and devices that help you to establish a routine of moving into a coherent heart rate variability, and you can learn how to recognize when you are in this state, for there is a physiological shift in your body.

HeartMath has researched the intelligence of the Heart and Heart coherence for over twenty-five years. In their book, *The HeartMath Solution,* they discuss what they call "core heart feelings," which help us to more easily experience and maintain Heart coherence, including, "love, compassion, nonjudgment, courage, patience, sincerity, forgiveness, appreciation, and care."[1] I refer to these as positive Heart impulses and add to this list: gratitude, innocent perception, trust, joy, and playfulness.*

Just a note that what I refer to as gratitude is called appreciation by HeartMath. I consider appreciation to be the act of honoring the beauty and gifts of someone else. For instance, telling a lover, "Your smile lights up my Heart." Or telling a friend, "Your laughter is the balm that I needed today." There is too little appreciation in this world. We tend to think that appreciation is a gift we give someone else. However, since appreciation is a positive Heart impulse, it is also a gift we give to ourselves. In other words, when we tell a stranger, "Hey! I love those shoes," we give them a boost of Love and we feed our own Heart, helping us to stay in Heart coherence. Appreciation is also an important aspect to having a healthy and wonderful relationship.

Gratitude

Positive Heart impulses are important when we are communicating with Plants. We will discuss them throughout this book. Gratitude is essential for Plant communication. Gratitude is a magic wand, helping us to shift from the mundane or the horrible to the wondrous or even blissful. Gratitude allows us to quickly access our Heart intelligence. Plus, it is simple, accessible, and free.

If you want to experience your Heart center, say or think about what you are grateful for. Keep doing this until you feel a physical shift of your body relaxing. If you are distracted or upset, you may find this more difficult. Sometimes we think, "I don't have anything to be grateful for." This is just our brain and our conditioning talking. In truth, all of our lives are surrounded by blessings. If you are struggling to think of something, then I suggest beginning with the sky above, the ground below,

---

*I learned the term "positive Heart impulses" from Pam Montgomery.

gravity, air to breathe, food to eat, water to drink, the birds singing. Hopefully, this will give you momentum and you will soon be on a roll.

When you are having a good day, take a few minutes to write down what you are grateful for. Maybe you write ten things or maybe it's one hundred. Keep this list with you. The next time you want to move into Heart coherence, read the list. Read it when you're having a bad day or an argument with a loved one or aren't feeling well, and notice the effects.

As you express what you are grateful for, you may notice physical changes. How is your body responding? You may notice that your body relaxes or your breathing slows. For me, my shoulders drop (sometimes several inches), my breathing slows and deepens, I feel that my Heart is huge and open, and my body feels puffy. My hands and feet especially feel large, like I am wearing Mickey Mouse's gloves and clown shoes. I am calmer and happier. When I feel this, I know that I am experiencing Heart coherence.

Once you are in your Heart center, you can ask a question or explore a "problem." You may want to write. Some prefer to do stream of con-sciousness writing during this time—writing with the nondominant hand, continually moving the pencil, writing down whatever words or thoughts come to mind, not paying attention to or judging them. You might be surprised by what comes to you. Often the best solutions are quite simple.

Gratitude is an incredible skill that can change our lives. I once had a root canal. I cannot take epinephrine and the endodontist was concerned that the pain medicine wouldn't last through the procedure. Before we started, I focused on gratitude and continued throughout. Rather than the horrible experience I was expecting, my root canal was blissful with no pain! Even the endodontist and nurse looked blissed out and a little surprised when we were finished.

My students and clients get tired of my recommendation of focus-ing on gratitude. Even though they have each experienced the magic of this, they are caught in the conditioning that it's too simple. Humans are a funny bunch. Everyone wants a magic pill to make their "prob-lems" disappear. And yet when you offer them a simple solution that actually works, they discount it because it's too easy—they have to suffer in order for something to be of value. The truth is that gratitude is that magic pill or, as I prefer, magic wand. The happiest people are not those with lots of money, fancy cars, and houses. The happiest people are those whose lives are based on gratitude, for their entire lives (no matter how challenging) are surrounded by gifts.

Whenever I think of gratitude, I think of my friend Phillip. Phillip worked in our local market. I never saw him without a beaming smile on his face. Over the years Phillip shared with me part of his story, which was filled with challenges and trauma. But none of his struggles stopped him; in fact, they added to his joy. Whenever I saw him, I'd ask how he was doing and he would say the same thing: "I'm great! I woke up! I'm alive! Life is goooood!" (I wish you could hear his voice, as that is what adds the real magic to his words.) He added such beauty to my life. When I was having rough days, his gratitude was infectious and transformed my day. Phillip died suddenly a few years ago. An eclectic group of people packed the church for his funeral. All of them shared the same story of Phillip: his smile, his laugh, his kindness, and his incredible love of life. He knew that the secret to a happy life was gratitude.

I have heard people say that gratitude can be a toxic trait designed to shame people who are suffering or encourage people to ignore their feelings. Shame is not part of the journey with Plants. Plants do not use shame or guilt or "not enoughs." These are human creations. Plants encourage us to live our authentic Truth, which means experiencing all of our emotions. Embracing gratitude does not mean pasting a fake smile on and ignoring our problems. But if we can access gratitude when we are in the midst of a problem, we may find that our suffering is reduced.

Gratitude shifts our perspective by moving us into Heart coherence. This is the first step in consciously communicating with Plants. In other words, start listing what you are grateful for and look for your physiological shift. Once you are in your Heart space, the Plants will tune themselves to your frequencies, facilitating the communication process. Not only are we more easily able to communicate with Plants when we are in our Heart space, our communications are also more accurate, often bypassing our limiting beliefs or frameworks. Gratitude opens the doors into the magical world of Plants.

Innocent Perception

While engaging with Plants, it is important to remember the positive Heart impulse of innocent perception. Often we act as if everything that could possibly be known is known. The truth is that this is impossible. Everything, including the Plants and ourselves, is continually evolving. Innocent perception allows us to interact with a Plant as if this is the first time we are experiencing them, with eyes of wonder, like children do. When we utilize innocent perception to engage with a Plant, our encounter is free of expectation or judgment, which assists us in receiving more accurate information. Judgment closes the Heart and limits our experience to a confined possibility. Innocent perception helps our interaction with the Plant be more enjoyable and fruitful.

Aren't we constantly learning more about our partners or close friends? We wouldn't view or treat them as if they were stagnant, without anything left to learn or give, nor would we want to think of ourselves that way. Life would be boring. Innocent perception allows each experience to be an opportunity for magic.

Common Concerns

Before we begin our journey with Plants, let's address some common concerns regarding Plant communication. The first is "What if people see me?" My response is always, "Great, let them see you!" But I understand the concern about people thinking it is weird to talk with a Plant. For some, this triggers an old fear of not wanting to seem too different from the predominant culture. Or there might be a fear of attracting attention. I have witnessed that most people have no awareness that I am communicating with a Plant or doing something "strange." They tend to walk right past me and my Plant friend. If you continue to communicate with Plants in public places, eventually some people will stop.

They may ask what you are doing or strike up a conversation or make a random comment. These people often need to hear about the potential of communicating with Plants. It is not uncommon for someone to respond, "I used to talk to Plants when I was a child." Sometimes I can see that I planted a seed for them, their eyes lighting up. Their random comment or even our conversation may offer information on the Plant's gift. Of course, if you are concerned, you can always say that you are resting or writing. But I have found that people need to witness the possibility of communicating with Plants and that when I can stand in the Truth of who I am and my wholeness, I invite others to do the same.

Plus, I think that it is weird to not communicate with other species. If we look back over the course of humanity, the true outliers are those who believe that we are separate from Nature and do not communicate with our other relatives. Imagine going to a large family reunion and ignoring all of your relatives except for your parents, not only refusing to engage in conversation with them, but acting as if they do not exist. This is the equivalent of what occurs every day when we do not engage with Plants, animals, and our other more-than-human relatives.

Another common concern is "What if I'm making this up?" My response again is "Great!" My friend Marjorie tells me that nothing is real, everything is made up. I remember this sometimes and it gives me permission to simply experience. There will be a time where we will use discernment, but for most of our process, we want to be open to all possibilities. If you like mysteries, you can think of yourself as Sherlock Holmes. We want to be exceptionally observant, taking note of everything, including our internal thoughts and emotions as well as the external environment. Sometimes we will think something and suddenly the wind will blow or the Sun will beam on us or a bird will sing—often, these are confirmations.

We will engage with the Plants with different techniques, each giving us another point of view, another opportunity to observe and "listen." During these exercises, we are simply noticing. Eventually we will review our observations, looking for patterns and meaning while we extrapolate our Plant's story; this is when we utilize discernment. We may notice some experiences that do not seem to fit the overall story or we may discover something that seems like too big of a stretch for us to confidently say that it is one of the Plant's gifts. (For example, perhaps you hear a message about treating cancer with your Plant, who is poisonous.) In those cases, we put a question mark by our observations and, if possible, do further research. Often you will find confirmation, but sometimes it can take years until a study is released or someone else receives the same information. Generally, we confirm the gifts of our Plant ally by working with them and noticing the effects. It is important to note that there are many ways to work with a Plant that do not include ingesting them, and we will talk about some of these throughout the book. I tend to err on the side of caution. If something doesn't feel safe to me, I don't do it. Trust your inner guidance.

The more you communicate with Plants, the easier it becomes to differentiate the Plant's voice or message from your own. I notice that the Plants generally phrase something differently than I would or the tone of the message is different than my typical internal thoughts. In time, you will discover how you tend to receive the Plants' messages. One of my students tends to receive poems, another songs, while some receive symbols. When these come in, they know that a Plant is trying to tell them something. There are different methods, and you will find the ones that are more comfortable for you. I generally sit and observe and then have a conversation with a Plant. But if there is something that I'm not clear about or if I want more information, I'll do a journey. There is no one right way to communicate with Plants, and it is best to engage with no expectations, even if you are a confident Plant communicator.

When I discuss Plant communication, people often wonder if I work with psychotropic Plants. Hopefully your experiences throughout this book will demonstrate that we are able to directly communicate with any Plant without the need for mind-altering substances. For centuries, people have utilized the gifts of psychotropic Plants to open their mind and Heart and help them experience other realms or gain wisdom or healing. Coming from a family with addiction issues, I was never attracted to psychotropics and have found that they are not necessary to communicate with Nature. I have had countless incredible, beautiful, conscious, and Heart expanding experiences with Plants without ingesting anything. I share some of these experiences and the lessons that I learned from them throughout this book.

Psychotropic Plants, like all Plants, have incredible gifts and are able to help humanity to heal and evolve. They are powerful teachers; one of their main lessons is the importance of Integrity (see chapter 4). Trauma and drama can occur when we engage with them through amnesiac consumption (including addiction, bliss seeking, and spiritual bypassing). People go to great lengths and money to experience these psychotropics, sometimes wearing the ceremonies like badges, often without contemplating the cultural and environmental implications. I have worked with numerous clients who have had psychotic breaks or experienced intense malevolent magic due to their experiences with psychotropic Plants (or the people facilitating the ceremonies). Therefore I generally caution people about engaging with them. We need to be mindful of the way in which we engage with a Plant as well as our intention, especially with psychotropics.

It is possible to work with these Plants, receiving their healings and learning their lessons, without ingesting them. While there is great research being done on the healing capabilities of psychotropics, it is important to remember that we can experience great healing and transformation with any Plant. The most important Plant for you is the Plant who is calling you. Humanity has long been out of alignment with Nature. It is time for us to engage in a respectful, reverent relationship with our kin.

One final note is that I ask people to refrain from consuming alcohol during Plant communication weekends. Alcohol is a depressant and, as such, it reduces our sensitivities. We rely heavily on our senses and intuition when communicating with Plants; this is not a time for diminishing their capabilities. I try to create a situation where my students are most likely to communicate with their Plant ally and therefore, we refrain from alcohol. While this is your process and you are free to choose, omitting alcohol is something to take into consideration.

Exercise: Accessing Your Heart Space

Moving into your Heart space and knowing when you are there is the basis for all of our work with Plants. We always want to be in our Heart space when we connect with Plants, allowing us to be more receptive and reducing the interference of our limiting beliefs.

- Find a quiet space where you can sit or lie down. You can also walk if movement is helpful for you.
- Close your eyes and take three deep breaths.
- List at least ten things that you are grateful for. If you find this difficult, then consider the sky above, the ground below, the breath of life, a time someone made you smile, the birds singing, the Plants, a food you love . . .
- Continue to list what you are grateful for until you feel a physical shift.
- Notice how your body feels. Are you relaxed? Has your breathing slowed? If so, you are in your Heart space or Heart coherence.
- What else do you notice about your body? Have your shoulders or neck relaxed? How does your Heart feel? Do you feel grounded and calm?
- You may want to repeat this exercise several times until you develop a clear sense of your body's reactions. These are the sensations that you are looking for whenever I refer to moving into your Heart space or Heart coherence in future exercises.

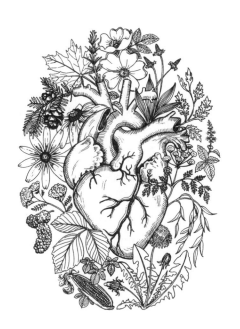

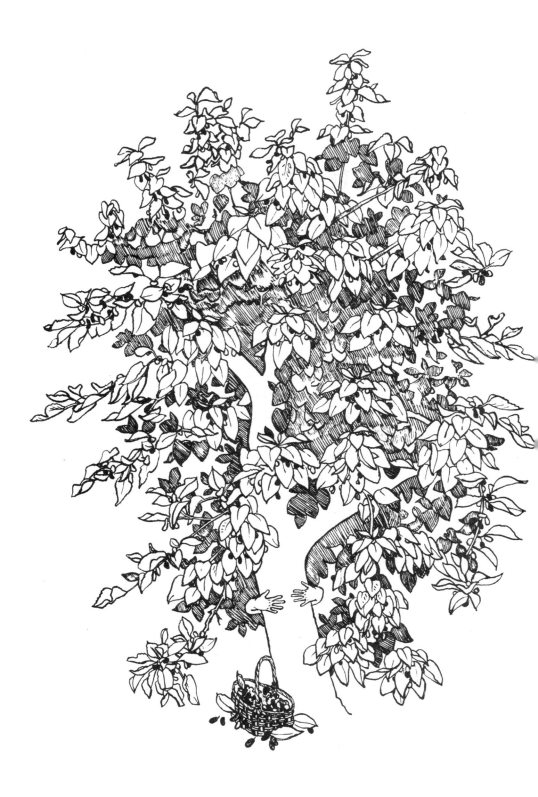

2

ᥰ Taste the Wild ᥰ
Mulberry

I believe my journey with Plant communication began with
Mulberry—although it may have started before I could even imagine. Do we ever really know when a journey begins?

I wake with the sun, listening to the birds sing. I quickly grab my basket and sneak outside while the house is quiet. This is my private time of
the day, a prized treasure when no one requires my attention. I prefer to
spend this time with the Plants. Today, I gather Mulberries for breakfast.

While I harvest, I process whatever is weighing on my Heart and any
decisions that I need to make. Sometimes, when I come out here, I am
quite weary, exhausted though the day has just begun. Within moments
of picking, my inner child comes out to play. I feel lighter and have more
energy. Soon, I'm starting to see the solutions for my problems, or maybe
that they aren't problems at all but opportunities. I head back to the
house with a full basket and calm Heart, ready to start my day.

This was before I thought I was able to communicate with Plants.
And yet, Mulberry was communicating with me. I learned much from
my mornings with ki. It was Mulberry who first asked me to write
a book.

Since I was a child, Mulberry has had a special tug on my Heart. I
climbed ki's branches to harvest berries, eating while I was gathering. I

sold these at a little stand I set up in front of my grandparents' home. I was happy to see that others enjoyed these treats too. Later, my grandmother told me, "People bought the Mulberries because they felt sorry for you." I don't believe her. I think about my children and their friends who come in dripping purple with enormous (purple toothed) smiles, some with bellyaches from eating too many berries and some who do not want to leave because they want more. I've seen the glimmer in the eyes of those who eat Mulberries. And I know the many "lost" mornings I have had as I wanted to eat just one more.

There is something about Mulberry that speaks to our innate Wild Self and allows our inner child to radiate. Perhaps it is the innocence and sweetness of harvesting and eating a wild food rarely found in stores. It is as if this tiny purple berry contains the secrets of the universe. (I think perhaps ki does.)

Mulberry helps us remember the pleasure that this world so abundantly offers. As we nibble on a berry, perhaps our own love affair with Nature begins. I delight in introducing people to Mulberry and witnessing their faces transform with joy and ecstasy, amazed that they can eat a berry off a Tree. Perhaps this is the greatest gift that Mulberry offers, to help us fall in Love with Nature.

Loving Nature

I want us to *absolutely* love Nature. This is the real revolution. This is how we "save" the Earth. This is how we save ourselves.

When we love someone, we recognize their value, we want them to succeed and be healthy. We enter into courtship and honoring, rather than wondering what is in it for us. Therefore it makes sense that if we want to help heal the Earth, if we want to shift climate change, we need to love the Earth.

In truth, the Earth does not need us to heal. When we talk about healing the Earth, we mean creating a place that is habitable for humans. For me, loving Nature is about more than this. Loving Nature is about shifting our perspective and recognizing the incredible beauty that surrounds us. Loving Nature is about gratitude for the abundance of gifts and support Nature generously provides. Loving Nature includes loving humanity. Loving Nature is about honoring *all* life. Ultimately loving Nature is about loving ourselves, for we are part of Nature. When we truly love Nature, we realize that we are surrounded by Love. We are connected to all. We are never alone.

As we hear stories of Earth's "destruction" and changes, it can be easy to fall into despair and hopelessness. This is when we need to take the time to go back to Nature and look, listen, and experience. When we do this Nature guides us. Nature does not say that all is lost or that humans are awful. Nature reminds us of who we truly are and helps bring us back into alignment with all of creation. As I sit with the Nature Spirits, they tell me to plant Trees or to clean out an area or show me how to slow run-off from flowing into the creek. Nature tells me that the changes are okay, that, in fact, change is the constant of Nature. I prefer to listen to Nature rather than the scientists who give the bleak reports.

I am not advocating that we do nothing, for that is definitely not what Nature wants. Nature wants us to engage and connect. Love is a verb—it requires attention and action. Nature wants us to utilize our incredible bodies to create beauty and health. Nature wants us to come back into rightful relationship with her. Nature wants us to realize that we are Love(d).

Multiple Perspectives

It is this Love (and patience) that I experience as I gather my breakfast. I no longer climb the Trees to harvest berries. Instead, I stretch and bend sometimes in amazing angles, surprising myself. Who needs yoga when you have Mulberry! I pull branches down low and occasionally jump up when Mulberry challenges me, leaving the higher berries for the birds (or perhaps the birds leave the lower berries for me).

As I do this, Mulberry asks if I found all the berries on a branch. I am confident that I have. However, Mulberry tells me to look again.

So I change my perspective and discover ten berries that I missed. We sometimes repeat this again and again while I stand in the same area, simply shifting my perspective and discovering more deliciousness. It seems no matter how many different perspectives I try, Mulberry tells me to look again and sure enough, there are berries.

Mulberry is teaching me about the importance of multiple perspectives. We live within a culture of dichotomies. We talk about opposites: good and bad, black and white, rich and poor, sick and healthy, young and old, friend and enemy. However, this is an illusion. The Plants do not live in this reality. They are able to see that what we think of as bad or evil can be flipped around and, from another perspective, can be considered good.

How many times have you shared an experience with someone but when you hear them tell the story of what happened, you think, "That's not at all what occurred!" Or maybe you have a conversation and later someone says what you told them and you say, "I didn't say that!" or "That's not what I meant." It doesn't really matter, because that is what happened in their reality. I experienced this a lot while raising my children. I'm sure you can relate to getting two different stories in response to the question, "What happened?" (That is, if it is not the common response of "I don't know.")

One example is how my youngest son and I remembered the time his second grade class hatched chickens. We agreed to take three chickens (having already experienced a disaster raising chickens on our farm). I asked for three hens, but apparently sexing chicks is not a skill set that is taught to second grade teachers, for we ended up with two roosters and one hen. The chicken coop was about fifteen feet from my bedroom window. If you've never raised chickens, let me say that the belief that they crow when the sun rises is a myth. Ours started crowing around 3 a.m.! Even worse, the hen was so confused that she also started crowing, and not very well.

After months of early morning crowing, the hen started to lay eggs. One night my son forgot to close the door to the coop, and we came out the next morning to a dead hen (we had only gathered two eggs). So now we had two roosters, which was not what I wanted. We asked my youngest what he wanted to do, giving him several options. Meanwhile, every night I hoped he would forget to shut the door again. Two nights later, he did and a raccoon killed one of the roosters. One left. We again asked him what he wanted to do, saying it wasn't very fair to the rooster to be all alone. (I should note that I had been a vegetarian for seventeen years and my kids had been vegetarians from birth. We had only started to eat meat two years prior to this.) After thinking for days, he came to us on a Sunday afternoon and said he wanted to butcher the chicken. Fortunately, my then husband had already taken a butchering class, so we quickly went into action before our son could change his mind.

This is where our stories differ. For me, what happened was horrifying. My husband did not sharpen the ax. He put the chicken on a large log we had and tried to chop off the head. However, the ax rebounded and he did not cut through. I won't go into more detail; I'll just say that it took many times before he was finally able to kill the chicken. We then completed the process of preparing the chicken to eat, to end up with about half a cup of meat (I was the only one who actually ate it).

Years later, I was talking with my son and he asked me if I remembered that day. I said yes, preparing to hear how traumatic it was for him. However, what he said was quite the opposite. He remembered that the chicken laid out his head on the log, offering his life.

To me this was a horrifying experience, and to my son, it was beautiful. Both are true.

As humans, we tend to be myopic, thinking our experience is the only true one or even the most important. We also have limited physical vision. To test this, stretch your arms out, lifting them to shoulder height. While facing forward, how far can you open your arms out to the sides and still see both of your hands? This is the range of your vision. While it is possible to broaden this range, we are able to see more of someone else's environment than we can of our own, both physically and metaphorically. To me, this is why it is important to work in community; together, we have a more complete picture.

Mulberry's lessons on shifting my perspective have been helpful in my life. I feel that this has helped me to be a more compassionate and understanding person. The current culture has us divide into factions based on our beliefs, appearance, nationality, diets, and so on, which supports and reinforces the myth of separation. I once heard that we commit an act of violence every time we label someone, for we create a wall that separates us. It is easy to write people off as "others." And yet, if we are to have peace and if we are to live up to our potential to love, we need to recognize that we are not as different from one another as we think. There are times that this is easy, that we can find commonalities across cultures, for example. But what about when you meet someone with completely different ideologies? What about when you meet someone who is a racist? Or the CEO of a gas company putting a pipeline in your community? Can you find the connection then?

Mulberry has shown me that I must continue to look until I can get a more accurate picture of the person and the situation. Until I can find the connection, understand the beliefs or actions, or recognize an underlying wound or trauma. This does not mean that I have to agree with them, though. Simply—can I understand why they do what they are doing, knowing that if I had the same life experiences as them, I would most likely have the same beliefs? And then, can I find a way to feel Love?

Love is the ultimate catalyst. When we can love someone, we open the doors of possibility. Maybe nothing changes (or seems to change). Though it's also possible that Love allows the person to have a change of Heart. Many experiments have shown that the thoughts and emotions of those around us affect us. The story of the Weissers, a Jewish couple who received threats from a KKK grand dragon, is one of the most memorable stories I've heard. Instead of getting angry at him or ignoring him or pressing charges, they wrote him letters with passages from Proverbs. They called him and offered to help him with his groceries. Eventually, he resigned from the Klan, wrote apologies, and converted to Judaism. When his health was failing and he didn't have long to live, he moved in with the Weissers, who took care of him until his death. This is the power of Love. (Their story is told in the book *Not by the Sword,* written by Kathryn Watterson.)

It would have been understandable for the Weissers to respond with anger toward this man or to write him off as evil. However, as Mulberry asks us to do, they looked from a different perspective and saw that this was a man who was hurting and angry and needed compassion and Love. I don't believe that they intended to convert him to Judaism and I'm sure they didn't expect that they would live with him. They simply saw that there was more to this story than hate and evil. Imagine what this world could be like if we responded more frequently with Love.

Mulberry shows me that finding solutions can be a rather tasty adventure. Perhaps all we need to do to find common ground is to share some wild food together and enjoy the sweetness of Mulberry.

The Unique Gift of Trees

It is not surprising that the Plant who opened me to Plant communication is a Tree. Trees capture our imagination and our Hearts, perhaps because they can tower over us and take many different forms or perhaps because they can outlive several generations. Trees play a pivotal role in art, history, and mythology. Many cultures have a special Tree that they consider to be the Tree of Life. For the Maya, this is the Ceiba Tree. The World Tree for the Norse was the Yggdrasil, an Ash. The Druids' Tree of Life is the Oak. These Trees connect the Earth and the cosmos or heavens. They also connect the present with the past, including the Ancestors.

Trees help to hold the memory of a Landscape. When we connect with them, we have access to the events that occurred in a specific area. Walking into a Redwood Forest feels like walking back in time; these Trees contain the memory of life before colonization. They hold the imprint of a time when humans lived in harmony with Nature. We can sense this and are awakened to the magical possibility.

In my practice, I have noticed that people who experienced a traumatic childhood, including living in an unloving home, and yet managed to become relatively healthy and intact adults often had a special Tree friend. They were able to find safety with their Tree friend and would visit ki or hide among ki's branches whenever the situation was over-whelming. It appears as if their Tree friend helped them to survive and even thrive, providing the Love and nurturing relationship they needed.

Bessel van der Kolk says, ". . . it's possible to survive just about any-thing, as long as you have—the people who are important to you are on your side."[1] I suggest that a Tree friend can fulfill this important role, acting as a loved one who is on your side.

I regularly suggest that my clients spend time with Trees. Sometimes this is to help them with anxiety or grief or to simply ease the transition from work to home. Simply being with a Tree helps to strengthen our etheric forces, calming our nervous system, bringing us into the present moment, and shifting us into Heart coherence. When someone experi-ences a sudden shock or trauma, I encourage them to spend as much time with Trees as possible. The Trees help them to come back into their body and lessen the energetic effects of the trauma. Trees are able to absorb and transmute the energies that are too large for us to carry.

This is an incredible gift that the Trees offer us and yet, if a large trauma like a massacre or fire continues to energetically affect an area long after the event, the Trees might be anchoring the energy of the trauma in the Land. In this case, we may need to help the Trees to heal and release the traumatic energies that they hold, so that the Land and the Beings who live there are no longer affected by these energies.

If we look at a Tree, we can see that they connect the Earth and the sky, helping us to do the same and to remember our own connection to the Earth and the cosmos. Kahlil Gibran writes, "Trees are poems that the earth writes upon the sky." Trees act like antennae anchoring the energy of the cosmos into the Earth and sharing the energy and messages of the Earth with the cosmos. They are our sentinels, guiding us through life.

There is an eco-society in Italy called Damanhur. This intentional community recognizes the intelligence of Nature. Trees play a vital role in the community. There are two practices from Damanhur that I share with my students. The first is that every nucleo (their co-housing units) has a welcoming Tree. Before entering the home, whether as a resident or visitor, you greet this Tree, generally placing your forehead on the trunk. This is a beautiful way of preparing to enter the house, helping to move into Heart coherence while also recognizing the protection that this Tree provides for the inhabitants. The second is that everyone has their special Tree. They are asked to choose a Tree with whom to enter into relationship. They meet with this Tree regularly and are responsible for ki's health and well-being. Given what I know about the connection between Trees and healing from trauma, I think everyone should have a special Tree. More than helping us to be healthy, this would encourage us to consider the well-being of our more-than-human kin.

When my children were young, we planted a Tree for each of them. We moved away several years later, but they found other Trees to connect with. We measured their growth with baby Poplar Trees who were soon beyond our reach. Some Trees were treasured for being great climbers, while others were great hiders. I love so many Trees. I have favorites around the world. And yet, I always keep an eye out for Mulberry Trees whenever I wander. If I see a Mulberry Tree somewhere, I know that there is magic and the Land wants to play and connect with humans. Mulberry welcomes me Home.

Exercise: The First Meeting

You are about to start a relationship with a Plant. Whether this is your first time or the hundredth, it is exciting!

Sometimes our traumas or beliefs that we are unworthy or unlovable can resurface. If that is the case, then know that this is an opportunity to heal for I guarantee that there is a Plant who wants to be in relationship with you. If you are willing, this Plant will show you that you are Love(d).

🌿 Take a walk. Who is calling you? Who has been trying to get your attention? Allow yourself to be called by a Plant.

🌿 There may be a Plant who keeps showing up in your life or maybe one that seems to be stunning. The Light might be shining on a certain Plant or perhaps it looks as if one is waving to you. You may think that a Plant is too obvious, that ki is so gorgeous and everyone is noticing ki. I assure you this is not true; the Plant is trying to get your attention.

- You may also find many Plants calling to you. Plants are always communicating with us. When they discover that someone wants to communicate, they get excited, which can overwhelm the human. If this is your experience, thank them and remind them that you can only work with one Plant at a time. And then ask, who is the Plant for you to connect with today?

- If you have any doubt, close your eyes, take several deep breaths, start listing what you are grateful for until you feel the shift into your Heart. With your eyes closed, feel the direction your Heart wants to move toward. Follow your Heart.

- It is possible that when you go to where you were called you do not feel a strong connection with the Plant, particularly if you were called by a Tree. If this is the case, look around the area, there may be a smaller Plant who wants to work with you.

- Don't worry, you can't do this wrong!

- Now that you've been called to a Plant, introduce yourself.

- Begin to breathe with the Plant. Become conscious of the fact that you are breathing in the Plant's exhale and ki is breathing in your exhale. Feel this exchange. Recognize that you are receiving a gift and offering a gift to the Plant. Now breathe in the Love from the Plant and exhale your Love to the Plant.

- Feel the innate connection and Love between you. This Plant wants a relationship with you. How does that feel?

- When you are finished, thank the Plant.

- Congratulations, you met and communicated with a Plant ally! Enjoy this moment.

- There is a tendency to want to research the Plant or identify ki if you do not know who they are. I encourage you to stay in the not-knowing and trust the development of your relationship. There will be a time for researching the information that others share about this Plant. Let's first discover what the Plant wants to share with you.

- If you do not know who this Plant is, you can ask them what they would like to be called. Many of the names, particularly the scientific names, have been created by dead White men. While it is helpful to have a common language to discuss Plants, we can let the Plants tell us what they prefer to be called. When I make Essences as I travel, I often do not know who a Plant is. One Plant told me that their name is Beauty Plant. I later learned that this Plant is known as Torch Ginger, though my Essence is still called Beauty Plant for this is truly who the Plant is.

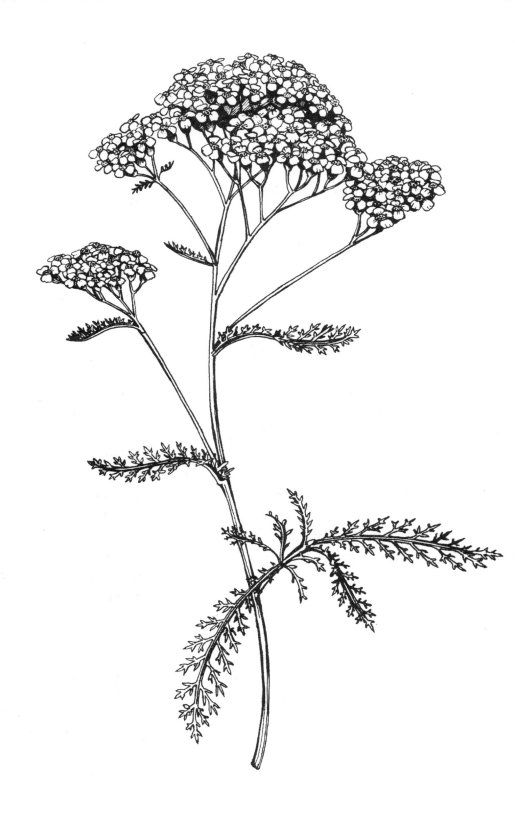

3

✑ New Opportunity ✑
Yarrow

For as long as I can remember I have been interested in natural healing. Growing up, Aloe was a regular in our house. My mom doesn't enjoy gardening; however, she has the most beautiful house Plants. When my house Plants are struggling, I send them to her for healing. For my mom, a house is not complete without Aloe. She taught me to put Aloe on burns. I was comforted in the knowledge that I could get relief from our beloved house Plant, which seemed like pure magic. My grandparents taught that food is medicine and the best, healthiest food comes from your garden. I remember Parsley was a favorite medicine of my paternal grandparents. Eating Parsley was a cure-all. They dried large amounts every year. As a teenager, I wasn't quite sure what I was supposed to do with the jars of dried Parsley they gave me. Though for them, they were giving me a jar of Love and their secret for a long, healthy life. (They both were active and healthy well into their nineties and lived to be 99 and 100 years old.)

When I was in sixth grade, I learned that Thyme tea with a little honey was good for bronchitis. I came down with bronchitis two years in a row. I never liked taking medicine (the notorious story is how it took four adults—my parents and paternal grandparents—to hold me down to get me to take my medicine). The pseudo-grape amoxicillin that I was given for the bronchitis was the worst. I was ecstatic when Thyme tea worked!

I was hooked; I wanted to learn all that I could about herbs and healing with Plants. In junior high, I learned about Flower Essences and homeopathy. In college, when people got sick, they came to me for help, which was often simply a cup of tea or warm soup and Love. Still, they felt better. I think that is where I learned that sometimes the most healing and loving act we can do for a person is to sit with them and listen to them.

My children came into my life when I was young. They became my focus, my reason for existence. I did not want to give them antibiotics and so my interest in herbs became more serious. Trying to keep a family healthy is one of the best ways to learn about herbs (though my children might disagree). It enables you to experiment and get creative, as well as learn herbs and techniques that truly work. Who wants to waste time on a possible remedy when your child is having a croup attack at two in the morning?

Yarrow became an important Plant in our family. While I always have an Aloe plant in my house, as far as I'm concerned, my Home is not complete unless Yarrow is growing outside of it.

The Plant world amazes me. There are Plants who are about the size of a grain of rice (*Wolffia spp.*) and as large as the towering giants like the Redwoods or even Pando, the clonal colony of Quaking Aspen who covers over a hundred acres. Can you comprehend this, a Plant is as large as 100 acres? Their colors are astounding. In spring, the Virginia Bluebells bloom and I swear they turn the air blue at one of my favorite trails. Then there's the magical Ghost Pipe who is seemingly absent of color. The reds and fuchsias of Hibiscus, Dahlia, and Poppies overwhelm my camera and never photograph accurately. If you ever need a reminder that Spirit and Nature have a sense of humor, then look at the shapes of flowers, particularly Orchids. One of my favorites, *Anguloa uniflora,* looks like a baby swaddled in a cradle. There are Plants whose very clear resemblance to genitalia will cause one to blush and chuckle. Other Plants, like *Oncidium,* seem to be sprouting aliens. And their scents! One whiff of some sends me immediately into a state of bliss, such as: Stargazer Lily, Tulsi, Orange blossoms, and Jasmine. Others, such as the infamous Corpse flower, could make you retch. Of course, tasting Plants is one of life's great pleasures, from spices to Figs to Cacao to wild berries. But not all Plants are meant to be ingested—some, like Poison Hemlock can kill you fairly quickly. While there are deadly Plants, I believe that every Plant has healing gifts.

With such a wide and varied abundance of Plants it can be easy to focus on the showiest or the most exotic. Yet the simple, common Plants can be the most profound healers in our lives. It is rather difficult for me to refer to Yarrow as simple, for this Plant is a miraculous healer; however, for those who have not fallen under Yarrow's spell, you might easily overlook the feathery green leaves or even the umbels of tiny white blossoms who seem to glow in the moonlight. If Yarrow catches your eye, you might (mistakenly) think, "What a delicate Plant."

Yarrow is a styptic, meaning that ki stops bleeding. Yarrow saved us—my two very active sons, but also myself and visitors—from getting stitches on numerous occasions. The old saying is that Yarrow is for "cuts to the bone." I witnessed the truth of this.

Several years ago, I was trying to remove a patch of tall Grass from our small pond. I wrapped the Grass around my hand and pulled, ki did not come out; however, the Grass cut my thumb clear to the bone, blood was rushing everywhere. This was early evening on a Sunday and I did not want to go to the emergency room, nor did I want stitches. I asked Yarrow to help and started packing my wound with ki's leaves, which I replaced as they filled with blood. Within minutes the bleeding stopped. I did not need stitches, my wound healed quickly without any infection, and now I have only an almost imperceptible scar, which to me is a reminder of Yarrow's gifts. This is only one of many experiences where Yarrow helped us heal. There has not been a time that we asked Yarrow to help and ki did not stop the bleeding. Sometimes it has taken hours, like when my partner almost cut off the tip of his finger while making salsa, but Yarrow eventually succeeds.

When my oldest son was a child, he would get nosebleeds during the winter from the dry air. We again took advantage of Yarrow's styptic qualities, putting leaves up his nose, which quickly stopped the bleeding. When I planted my herb garden, Yarrow and three Elderberry Bushes were at the center of the spiral. I was grateful for the assurance of Yarrow's location on those freezing cold, middle of the night emergency harvests. And I was always grateful that Yarrow's effectiveness allowed me to quickly return to dreamland. (To be fair, my son did not always enjoy Yarrow's support because ki tickled the inside of his nose. But the nosebleeds stopped.)

Yarrow is also an incredible remedy for colds, flu, and fever. Here the key phrase is "chills to the bone." Yarrow and Elderflower tea have helped me many times. As soon as I feel that I'm coming down with the flu, I take a bath with a strong Yarrow tea. Again, the effects are amazing and I am grateful for some respite.

Protection

On an energetic level, Yarrow is a remarkable protector. Your aura is the protective field that surrounds you, which keeps out unwanted energies including negative thoughts and safeguards from overstimulation (which often leads to anxiety and eventually mental breakdown). We are energetic Beings who live in a sea of energy. If we could see what surrounds us, we would be overwhelmed. Your aura additionally keeps your Soul Force and vital energy harnessed within, allowing you to experience the full benefit of these, including feeling healthy, energized, and nourished. We can engage in situations or have experiences, however, that cause an energy leak—meaning our vital energy is seeping out of our aura. We may not notice it at first; however, if the leak grows or is compounded, we may feel tired. We say, "I feel drained." If the leak is sustained long enough or becomes a deluge, we may lose sense of who we are or feel as if we can no longer go on with life. It's important to notice what causes our energy leaks and to shift those behaviors so that we can again have full access to our energy and feel like our vital, healthy, sparkly selves. As you can see, our auras have a very important role in our lives. Various illnesses and dis-eases occur when our auras are not functioning properly.

Many actions that contribute to good health and physical hygiene also strengthen our auras: eating foods that support your body, getting enough sleep, meditation or other stress reducing activities, doing things that fill you up, unplugging (cell phones, Wi-Fi), moderate exercise, and spending time in Nature.

However, we often need more support to keep our auras strong. Fortunately, when there is a need, Nature provides an abundance of solutions. There are many great protector Plants, including Yarrow, St. John's Wort, Echinacea, Stinging Nettles, Motherwort, Angelica, Achiote (Annatto), Garlic, Rue, Marigold, Tulsi (Sacred Basil), Rosemary, Poison Ivy, and others. We will talk about some of these later in the book. Each Plant has their own style or flavor of protection. You may resonate more with a particular Plant, which is who you should work with for protection. Yarrow acts like a shield protecting our aura.

There are many ways in which we can work with these Plants for protection. We can plant them around our house, carry them with us, or make a spray with them to use on ourselves or in our spaces. We could ingest an Essence or, if they are not poisonous, a tincture or a tea. We can wear clothing that has an image of them on it or jewelry made from them. And we can simply ask them to surround us with protection.

While I think protection is important, becoming obsessed with protection is harmful. I compare this to washing our hands. Washing our hands is important, but if we spend hours scrubbing our hands until they are red and bleeding, we harm ourselves. When we get obsessed with protection, we cause an energy leak or draw to us the energies that we don't want.

When I need extra strength, I call on Yarrow. After my Pop-Pop died, I asked for Yarrow's support as I gave his eulogy. I put Yarrow in the pocket of my suit. I asked Yarrow to help me as I went through many contentious divorce meetings. Every time, I could feel Yarrow helping to hold me, protect me, and give me strength. Yarrow is always there waiting to help; we simply need to ask.

Door Opener

Yarrow's herbal qualities and protective actions are wonderful and are a good reason to have Yarrow growing near you. However, the real reason why Yarrow makes my home a Home is that it is Yarrow who offered me an opportunity to be in a conscious relationship with Nature. Actually, what ki said was that if I would like, ki was willing "to open the doors for me into the Plant world."

An incredibly challenging experience precipitated this offer from Yarrow. One winter morning, my son woke up with a heavy nosebleed. I immediately went outside to gather Yarrow, only to discover that ki was gone. The Elderberry Bushes were gone as well. I couldn't find them anywhere. (I later discovered a very tattered and torn Elderberry Bush nearby.) I was completely lost; my cherished friends were missing and I was unable to help my son.

I soon discovered that someone, who I think was well intentioned, had tried to help my garden get "back into shape." I have never been a pristine gardener and that year we were building our house, which meant that I had even less time to focus on the garden. In the process of their efforts to help, my garden was destroyed and the Plants disappeared. To say that I was shocked and heartbroken does not even come close to describing my feelings. Over the next several months, this person and I had many conversations that often led to large arguments and, ultimately, our relationship was ruined. This was a very difficult time for me; I lost my herb garden, my Beloveds, and I lost an important friendship. I also had my reality attacked and questioned. But in my Heart, I knew the truth. I had spent hundreds of mornings with these Plants; I knew this garden possibly better than I knew my own body, and I was not willing to ignore what happened nor to believe stories that were not in alignment with my experience.

It was after one of these conversations, where I again advocated for the Plants, that Yarrow presented me with this opportunity to go deeper into the Plant world. I didn't have to think twice. I immediately responded, "*Yes!*"

That day, I had no idea what exactly Yarrow meant nor did I know what this would look like and, really, I would never have been able to imagine the way in which my life has unfolded since that day. I simply knew that my Heart yearned to be in communion with the Green Beings and I trusted Yarrow. All these years later, I know I made the right choice and I am grateful for it. I now know that the gift Yarrow offered me was a relationship with the Plant Spirits. This gift (with other assistance) is what led me to study with Pam Montgomery and learn Plant Spirit Healing, as well as many other wonderful adventures with Plants. Saying yes to Yarrow greatly shifted my life and helped me to return to my Soul's path, for, in many ways, I had been lost.

Plants and Nature certainly appreciate when we speak and stand up for their rights. When they know that we are dedicated to them, no matter how imperfect we are, they are more willing to share their gifts with us. This makes sense, of course. Aren't we all more willing to share our gifts with people with whom we feel comfortable and safe?

While this is part of my story with the Plants, there are many ways to hear the calling or move into a more conscious relationship with Nature. Ideally, we don't need adversity to do this. The calling can be a whisper and can occur in many different forms. Perhaps there is a Plant who caught your eye and you want to know more about them. Perhaps you are experiencing an illness that the medical field cannot explain. Perhaps you love to draw Plants. Perhaps you are learning how to grow your own food, or you are helping a piece of Land heal. Perhaps you have been dreaming of Plants, maybe even some whom you have never seen before, or you remember how Plants were your friends when you were a child. Or perhaps there is a deep yearning inside of you. If you have been experiencing this calling, I encourage you to say "*Yes!*"

I have helped many people awaken to their call and move into a more conscious relationship with Plants. I know that this invitation is unique and there is something universal in it, a feeling that previously something was missing or that there was an emptiness. In all my years of guiding people through this process and all the many others I have met who have answered the invitation, I have never heard someone wish that they had said "no." Usually, people are in tears and say, "I wish I learned this earlier" or "Why did I wait so long?"

If you want to be in communion with Nature and are unsure that you have been invited, I can assure you that you have. For that is our birthright: we are Nature, we are meant to be in partnership with all of Nature. I encourage you to create an intention stating your desire to learn and to be in partnership with Plants and Nature. They will recognize your intention.

Trust

Mostly, what we need to do is pay attention and trust. Trust is an important aspect of being in co-creative partnership with Plants. When we trust, we send an enormous "*Yes!*" to the universe and the universe responds accordingly. Sadly, however, most of us have been taught to distrust.

This starts in early childhood, when we are told that what we are experiencing, witnessing, or feeling is not true. For example, you go to the doctor and they tell you "This won't hurt," and yet it does. When you cry, they say, "It doesn't hurt that much," denying your experience and teaching you that your feelings are wrong. Or perhaps you can hear your parents fighting and you feel scared, as the emotions and energy are overwhelming. Your parents respond that everything is okay. They may try to act as though it truly is, and yet, you know that it is not okay. But who are you supposed to believe, your parents or yourself? As adults, too, how many times have we been lied to, whether it is a partner who swears that they are faithful despite obvious signs that they are not, a company who promises us results that do not happen, or a boss who guarantees us a promotion that does not come? Throughout our lives, we are taught to doubt or ignore our instincts, our feelings, our experiences, and, therefore our understanding of the world. It is no wonder that many of us do not trust. Thankfully, we can shift this pattern.

Trusting allows us to regain our understanding of the world. We can begin by paying attention to our bodies. Our bodies innately know what is good and right for us; when we are in alignment with this, our energy is strengthened. This is the basis of muscle testing and dowsing.

It is easier to hear what our bodies are saying if we are in our Heart space. Here is a brief practice in listening to our bodies if you'd like to try: Find a quiet space, and simply breathe, paying attention to your breath. After you take a few breaths, begin saying or thinking of things that you are grateful for. When you feel your body relax, ask a question—for example, is it good for my body to eat a piece of chocolate now? Or, does this class benefit me? It is best to start with something simple. After asking your question, pay attention to your physical reaction. Do you light up, feel energized, or excited? If so, that is a yes. Or do you feel drained, heavy, or contracted? If so, that is a no. Kate Gilday calls this the ping/thud method. Do you ping—resonate higher, feel enlivened—or thud—feel depleted or heavy? Really, what we are asking is, "Is this in alignment with my Soul?" When we focus on what makes us come alive, what makes us sparkle, what is in alignment with our Soul, our lives change. This is the space we want to be in, what is referred to as "the flow." Innocent perception is a particularly important aspect to this. We all have conditioning as to what feels good or what adds to our lives, but that conditioning may not be in alignment with your Soul. But your Soul (and your body) knows the Truth. Ask yourself every time, "Does this enliven? Does this feed my Soul?" You may be making Love or eating the most delicious chocolate ever and yet it might not be enlivening at that moment. We too often say yes when our body is saying no. This is a waste of energy, which depletes us and prevents us from truly experiencing the gifts of life, including bliss.

Practicing this method is a good way to reclaim our innate wisdom and trust in our body and instincts. Of course, this also means that we need to then follow those instincts. If we get a feeling that we should turn left when we always turn right, do it. If we feel that we should stay away from a person who wants to talk to us in a bar, listen to your body, no matter what your friends say. Again, it is important that we are in our Heart space when we are listening and learning to trust. This helps to reduce the risk of responding out of fear or trauma.

It can be scary to trust. We tell ourselves we are stupid or foolish.

We can feel like the sky is falling or that it is hard to breathe. In *Through the Eyes of Love: Book One,* Michael J. Roads receives a message from Pan: "I say unto you, trust beyond trust. Trust when trusting seems hopeless and pointless. While you stand in the ashes of despair, trust. While your heart feels shattered and broken, trust. Trust will take you into realms you have not yet walked, and trust will reveal to you sights you have not seen. Trust."[1]

When we trust the information that we receive from Nature, we access the wisdom of the ages. Life becomes less of a struggle, for we have more resources available to us and we are no longer wasting our time and energy. That does not mean that everything is easy or enjoyable. Trusting may require that we make difficult changes in our lives. With enough practice, we know that these changes are for the best, no matter the immediate pain.

It is common for people who are remembering how to communicate with Plants to think that they fabricated the information they received. They will discredit this information, and then later, as they learn more about the Plant, they discover that what they received made sense. Doubt diffuses our energy and creates a power leak. If we doubt enough, we no longer will know what is right for us. We then give our power to others to tell us how we should live our lives, what we should wear, what we should eat, and so on, to the point of losing our sense of who we truly are.

Part of trusting is paying attention to the "First Voice." This First Voice is powerful. What is it that you first hear or how do you feel when you begin to sit with this Plant? Ask a question. What is the first response that you receive? The more we trust, the easier this becomes and the more our confidence grows. Remember, every time we trust, we send a positive energetic response to the universe.

When we pay attention to the First Voice, we save ourselves quite a lot of trouble. If we are meant to learn a lesson, we will continuously be presented with opportunities to learn it. Do we want to learn this the first time or the hundredth time? Having overlooked many learning opportunities only to have another arise in a more difficult way (the proverbial two-by-four to the head—in my case sometimes, an eight-by-eight), I suggest that we learn our lessons as soon as we can.

Sometimes we do not understand what the Plants are trying to tell us. Still, we can trust that we will have clarity when we are ready. Occasionally, it has taken me years to understand an experience with a Plant. Then one day, it all becomes clear.

I recently was reminded of a ceremony with Yarrow that was particularly challenging for me. I decided to review my journal to see if I could understand what occurred. I was single at the time and everyone who knew me knew that I yearned for my Beloved; you might say I was obsessed with finding them. During this ceremony, Yarrow energetically introduced me to my Beloved. Ki told me that "our joining together is to bring Love into the world." I saw how our union helps to heal the Sanctuary and the people who come here. I also experienced an important past life during this ceremony. I struggled through the experience. Even after I returned home, I continued to struggle for weeks. I experienced temperature dysregulation, nausea, and loss of appetite (which was very unusual for me).

Reading about these experiences now, I have a completely different perspective. I am currently living with my Beloved and it is true that having him here has helped to heal the Land and has added a new level of healing to my apprenticeships. Right before we began our romantic relationship, I had received a life-changing healing that was centered on the life that I saw with Yarrow. This healing allowed me to truly feel loved and to experience romantic Love. Now I know that my struggle during and after the ceremony was because I was resisting Yarrow's offering of healing the past life. Yarrow was trying to show me my "weak" area or the blockage that was keeping me from my Beloved. I didn't understand this and on a subconscious level I resisted the healing. Fortunately, I was given another opportunity to heal.

Achilles' Heel

As my experience demonstrates, Yarrow helps us to understand our weaknesses, our vulnerable parts. I was told a story that when Achilles was born, his mother, Thetis, was warned that he would die in battle. Knowing that Yarrow is a supreme protector and wound healer, Thetis dunked Achilles in a Yarrow bath. However, she was holding him by the ankle, so that became the one place on his body that was not protected, his weak spot—hence the phrase "Achilles' heel" and Yarrow's scientific name, *Achillea millefolium*.

When we know our vulnerabilities, we are better equipped to deal with life. We know where we need to focus our attention or what needs to be healed or even how to work with our strengths. This is another reason why Yarrow is a great protector.

Sometimes the lessons or healing opportunities with the Plants are subtle and it may take time for us to become aware of them. In our culture, bigger is often considered better. I see this belief play out in the herbal community as well sometimes. People want strong herbs that will create an undeniable, almost immediate effect. Sometimes these intense healing experiences can create more trauma or slow down our healing process. In the desire for bigger, we can overlook the capability of healing simply by sitting or spending time with a Plant.

Looking back to that time when I "lost" my garden, I realize that Yarrow gave me another gift. At that time in my life, I had great difficulty in saying no or expressing any thoughts that were not in agreement with what people wanted to hear, especially if I thought it could create conflict or upset someone. I thought it was best to keep the peace and make others happy. I didn't realize the great cost of this including my own happiness, nor did I understand that my acquiescence did not benefit anyone. Many of us are taught when we are young to be sweet and kind, to not rock the boat. We are trained peacemakers. For some, this is a matter of survival. For others, like myself, this behavior was rewarded. While I would smile and agree on a conscious level, there were times where I responded on a subconscious level. These responses were never pretty. Sometimes I would hoard my resentments of all the times I ignored my desires until they came flying out like Mentos dropped into a can of Coke. Other times, my response came out sideways; I would act out in a passive aggressive manner, perhaps saying something snide or telling a mutual friend how I actually felt.

Yarrow helped me to see that these behaviors were not in my best interest, nor was I doing anyone any favors by ignoring my needs. It truly was revolutionary to discover that I was supposed to express my needs and feelings. The best thing was for me to use my voice and speak my Truth, even if that meant upsetting someone. Of course, that doesn't mean being nasty or malicious, but kindness doesn't always come with a smile, and it definitely never comes with a fake one. Nor does it mean that people will be happy to receive what I need to express, but in the long run it is for the best. Yarrow gave me courage to stand in my Truth and reclaim my garden. I had to start from scratch again, even replacing the rocks and paths, but I created another herb garden, and that garden came to be a great solace for me. When we engage in a more conscious relationship with Plants, like every good relationship, there is a give and take. I thought I was helping Yarrow, and yet Yarrow was helping me.

Yarrow has many gifts to offer us, far beyond those I've described. There is one other gift, however, that I feel is important to share here regarding Yarrow's incredible wound-healing capabilities—which can even help us heal the wounds of patriarchy.

Healing the Wounds of Patriarchy

Let's be clear, patriarchy is an abomination that is completely out of alignment with Nature. The foundation of patriarchy is the belief that some Beings (cis-gendered men) are more superior than others. Despite humanity's best efforts to force it, Nature is not hierarchical. Any system that says that something or someone is superior or inferior will eventually collapse. Nature always has their way. Of course, through human eyes, it may take a long time for the collapse to occur and great harm can be done during that time.

Patriarchy has contributed to countless wounds in our society over generations. Many of these are so deeply ingrained that we consider them to be part of our culture and do not understand the violence and injustice that they perpetuate. Patriarchy does not just harm those who identify as women. The patriarchal system enforces a strict code as to who is deserving. Generally, this has been defined by one's level of "masculinity" or maleness. As we heal and unravel the beliefs and roots of patriarchy, we discover that the traits we have defined as "masculine" and "feminine" are not gender norms but cultural conditioning. In other words, those who were assigned male at birth (AMAB) are not inherently more powerful, smarter, stronger, more violent, less emotional, less talkative, more dominating, more driven, more athletic, less spiritual, more competitive, more rational, more rebellious, more courageous, more sexual, or bigger sports lovers than those who were assigned female at birth (AFAB). Similarly, those who were AFAB are not inherently more nurturing, kinder, more sensitive, more emotional, more talkative, weaker, more submissive, more compassionate, more relationship-oriented, more spiritual, less resilient, less intelligent, less talented, less charismatic, more loving, or better cooks than those who were AMAB. These are traits that were either reinforced or discouraged or things we simply were or were not taught.

I am grateful to all of the feminist, gender bending, Queer, Nonbinary, and Transgender folx, as well as anyone else who has been pushing the edges of our understanding around gender and gender roles. This expansion helps us all to live more authentic lives and to break free of patriarchy, for gender is one of its foundations. My hope is that as we shift away from the patriarchy and unravel the beliefs and conditioning that it supports, we will come to understand that we do not live in a binary world of small boxes. Instead, we live in a multidimensional, multifaceted world of infinite possibilities.

In order to achieve this, we need to do some work, including understanding how we are affected by the patriarchal system. To succeed in a patriarchal system, cis-gendered men must adhere to these "masculine" traits. Often this means ignoring or not developing their true selves and desires, essentially starving their Souls to maintain the status quo and robbing the world of their gifts. As bell hooks writes, "The first act of violence that patriarchy demands of males is not violence toward women. Instead patriarchy demands of all males that they engage in acts of psychic self-mutilation, that they kill off the emotional parts of themselves."[2]

The patriarchal system also requires men to treat women and those deemed not masculine enough as less than in order to participate in a power over dynamic. We observe this even among the jeers of young children, such as "sissy boy" or "you run like a girl." Again, this goes against the very basis of the universe. Whenever we treat someone, be they a woman, a person of color, an animal, or a Plant, as though they have less value than ourselves, we devalue ourselves and hurt our own Soul.

For those growing up as female, we are taught almost from birth that there is something wrong with us, we can never be enough, we will always be lacking, simply because we were AFAB. This is psychological warfare that can destroy a person's self-esteem and sense of self while again robbing the world of their beauty, talents, and incredible gifts. This also creates a culture of competition between other women and girls including the alienation of cliques, cutting one another down, and backstabbing. These actions strengthen the belief of the patriarchy and keep us from working together to create a world where everyone's talents and gifts are appreciated. This is definitely not to say that people who were AFAB have not made incredible contributions, but how much energy has been wasted by trying to overcome the conditioning of the patriarchy or even by trying to play by its rules? How many talents were never discovered because women were deemed less than, were forced into more traditional feminine roles, or had their work stolen by men in power?

Women promote patriarchal thinking by accepting men's bad behavior as normal. This occurs in many ways including a "boys will be boys" mentality, brushing off sexual harassment or even assault and abuse, or accepting and believing that men should not contribute their fair share of household duties. We also support this when we fawn over men for mediocrity or even subpar behavior. For example, I have witnessed women practically worshipping a man when he changes a diaper or watches his children for an evening, when that is the basic duty of any parent, and I have seen how often women will consider a man an expert when they themselves have more experience and know more about the subject than the man. (I have witnessed this quite a bit in the herbal community; I've even done it myself.) And it's not just heterosexual, cis women who are prone to this. This is the patriarchy at work in our unconscious actions. This may seem like I'm male-bashing (the perpetual charge against feminism); however, I see it more as male loving. For the patriarchy also keeps men from developing into their wholeness, robbing them of some of the greatest gifts of life. My brother could turn a diaper change into a thirty minute process. Once I went to see if everything was okay and witnessed him in a beautiful exchange of Love with his son. He was singing to him and talking with him and just adoring him. This "chore" gave him an opportunity to connect with his child. How many moments of connection and intimacy have men been deprived of for the sake of the patriarchy?

The people and institutions who seemingly benefitted from patriarchy and uphold this system have committed horrible acts of violence. The success of the patriarchal system demands domination and domination requires violence. The Witch hunts and domestic abuse are obvious examples of this violence. However, we have been trained to accept domination as a natural part of our lives whether from our parents, our teachers, our partners, our bosses, our religion, or our mentors. We often ignore the effects and the cost of living in a system of domination, including the lack of Love. We ignore the violence or assume that it is a natural part of life, when we are all harmed by the smallest act. The effects of these violent acts continue to be passed down through our bodies in the form of generational trauma and fear.

Healing the wounds of patriarchy requires the efforts and attention of each of us. We all were born into this system and we all have beliefs based on it. I was raised by a strong feminist who was raised by a strong feminist. Feminism was a given in my family. I was shocked to discover that I had sexist biases.* The more I learn and heal, the more I

---

*You can check your own biases using the website of Project Implicit, a nonprofit organization whose mission is to educate the public about bias through research into implicit social cognition.

understand how greatly patriarchy has impacted my beliefs and actions. Hopefully it is clear that no one benefits from this system.

The issue with a patriarchal society is not that men are in control, and therefore the antidote is for women to be in control. The issue is the power dynamic utilized in patriarchy, which is often called "power over." Power over is the belief that certain people are superior and therefore should have control over the masses. This group retains their power through domination, fear, and othering. They use their power for their own benefit often through the exploitation of others. This power dynamic allows us to devour the Earth, to pollute the very water we drink, to clear-cut Forests, to wipe out whole species simply for material gain. There is great absurdity in the fact that we knowingly destroy the very Beings who allow our lives to continue for some pieces of cloth or metal that someone once said had value. How is it that humans are supposed to be the most intelligent species?

Obviously, the power over paradigm is not in alignment with Nature. Therefore, Nature wants to help us heal from this and to remind us of another way of living together in harmony with all Beings. Healing from the wounds of patriarchy is particularly important because for millennia humans have been following a pattern where oppressed people become oppressors and inflicted their trauma onto others. This only perpetuates the power over dynamic and compounds our traumas. Of course, there are exceptions to this pattern.

Patriarchy does not serve our society nor our evolution, and thus it is coming to an end. Much of the turmoil we are witnessing is the result of fear as the system dissolves while some try to desperately hang onto it. If we truly want to experience peace and live in co-creative partnership with Nature, we need to heal these wounds. If we do not, the nasty head of oppression will rise again in a different form. Yarrow can help us. We can work with Yarrow Essence, do a shamanic journey with Yarrow asking to have these wounds healed (see chapter 13), or participate in a ceremony with Yarrow for this purpose. On top of helping us heal, Yarrow can show us a different way of being in this world where all Beings, human and more-than-human, are treated as Sacred, a place where we utilize power with and within rather than power over. In other words, Yarrow can help us to heal and live up to our potential.

There are other systems that utilize the power over dynamic and incorporate the belief that some people are superior to others, including white supremacy, capitalism, homophobia, and some religions. We often see these systems working together because they utilize this power dynamic and therefore tend to support one another. Once you start to heal and shift toward a power with dynamic, all of these systems begin to crumble. Therefore, we can enter this great healing from many different angles. We can get caught up in the arguments that we need to focus on feminism first or racism. Often it is not a choice of either-or but both-and. We can't shift these systems if we are perpetuating the oppression of someone else. The real focus is to remember that all Beings are Sacred and have a right to thrive, that we are all connected, and that what harms you also harms me. It is important to remember compassion, for ourselves and others, as we uncover the roots and wounds of these systems and begin our healing, for this can be a painful process. We may have times of fear, resistance, or overwhelm, which are understandable. We are undoing deeply ingrained patterns often without a clear understanding of how else to exist in this world. Fortunately, the Plants are here to support us on this journey. They know how to live together in harmony.

I have worked with Yarrow to heal the wounds of patriarchy so I know that ki helps with this. It is possible that ki can help with the healing from these other systems as well. When there is a need, Nature provides a solution. I am sure that there are many other Plants who can help us to heal and shift the power over dynamics. I am beginning to work with Apple for healing the wounds of patriarchy since the story of Eve has been one of the most powerful tools used to show that women are inherently sinful and need to be controlled. For the last several years, I have grown Cotton to help heal the wounds of slavery and racism. We have forced Nature to support our systems of domination against ki's will and therefore we need to make amends to the Plants as well. As we do this, we lessen the stranglehold of these systems.

Love Letter from Yarrow

Dear One,
It will be okay
I am here
Breathe deep
Let your walls down
You are safe
As you break
You expand
I will glue you together again
Bigger, better, brighter
Remember it is in your weakness
that you are strong
You are born of the stars
the dreams of your Ancestors
brought into this mortal body
Move past the illusion
Embrace your fullness
Stand naked in your Truth
Swim in the waters of your emotions
Love so fiercely, you dissolve
Open your wings
And fly

Exercise: The First Voice

- Join your Plant ally, bringing with you a journal or paper and something to write with. Make sure you are comfortable—you may want a mat or chair to sit on.
- Greet your Plant.
- Move into your Heart space through gratitude. Spend time simply being in your Heart space with your Plant, at least twenty minutes, though preferably an hour or more. If you get pulled out of your Heart space and start to focus on the tasks in your life, return to gratitude.

- During this time, simply listen and be open, allowing yourself to be extraordinarily observant.
- You may experience images, songs, or sensations. . . . Phrases or information may pop into your head.
- You may notice aspects of the Plant or the area around ki. How does your body feel when you sit with the Plant? What is happening around you?
- Write your observations down even if they seem silly or bizarre or you think that you are making them up. For now, we are simply observing and noting, gathering information, paying attention to the First Voice. We are not assigning meaning to any of it. Interpretation and understanding will come later; we will use our discernment then.
- Remember, we want to engage in innocent perception with nonjudgment. Whatever you are experiencing is part of your conversation with the Plant.
- When you are finished, be sure to offer your gratitude to your Plant ally.

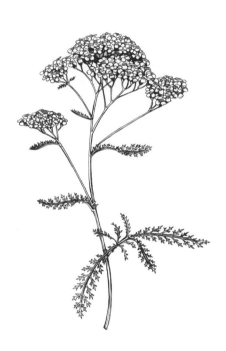

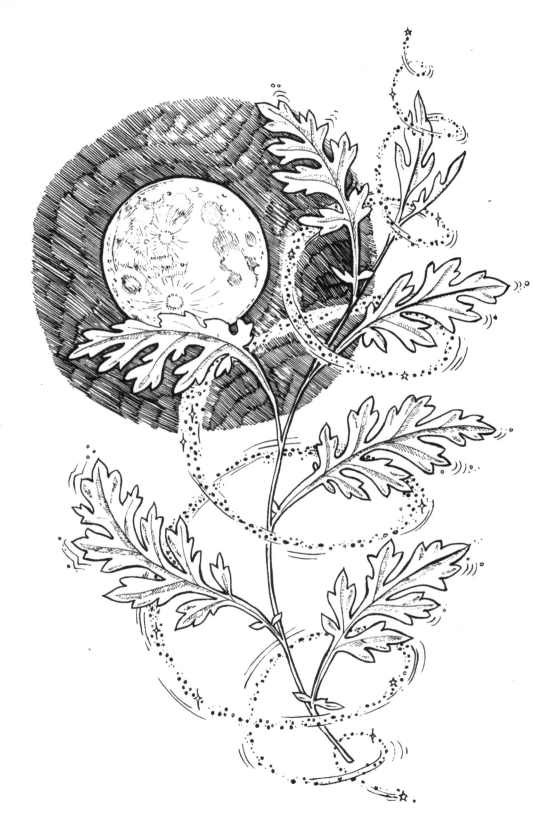

4

❧ Dare to Dream ❧
Mugwort

*I*met the Spirit of Mugwort during my Plant Spirit Healing
Apprenticeship with Pam Montgomery. It was a sunny day in June.
I sat with Mugwort on the banks of the stream at Sweetwater Sanctuary
in Danby, Vermont. As I sat there, I saw the Spirit of Mugwort as a
woman. Ki grabbed my hand, said, "Come with me," and led me down
the stream into the unknown. Since that moment, I have felt as if
Mugwort has been guiding me on an epic life journey.

> *The doorway to another World*
> *Begins with a green knob*
> *You open it wide*
> *I step through not knowing where we are going*
> *You do not even need to say*
> *"Trust me"*
> *For I do.*

Mugwort is one of the foundational Plants of Plant Spirit Healing
and HEARTransformation. Ki's Latin name is *Artemisia vulgaris*. Being
named after a Goddess is a significant indicator of this incredible Plant.
Artemis is a Moon Goddess and the Goddess of the Wild, never to be

domesticated. She is considered to be a "virgin" Goddess, meaning that she is whole unto herself. She is the Goddess of the hunt and childbirth.

Anyone who has met Mugwort knows that ki is not to be domesticated. *Artemisia vulgaris* is not native to the United States; however, ki is naturalized and quite generous. (*Artemisia douglasiana* is native to California and can be used interchangeably with *Artemisia vulgaris*.) When I moved to Heart Springs Sanctuary, Mugwort only grew along the road by the creek where the township mowed, so ki was quite straggly and never got tall. Fortunately, I have a friend who has an abundance of Mugwort that I could harvest. I laughed every time I pulled into his driveway. Mugwort grew sideways out of the brick retaining wall next to my car. Mugwort grew out of the cracks in his patio. The garden beds were filled with Mugwort. Everywhere you looked, Mugwort was growing. My friend was overwhelmed; I was grateful and in awe.

When I was studying herbs, I volunteered in the gardens of a local herbalist. I felt like the majority of my time was spent wrestling with wild Morning Glory and Mugwort. We pulled out more Mugwort than we could use. This left a large imprint. When I designed my first herb garden at the farm, I didn't include Mugwort. Over time, I missed having ki around. I was taught that before most people could read, Mugwort signified a healer—they might have a sign with a picture of Mugwort or ki might grow by the front door. One day I asked Mugwort to come to the farm. It should be noted that we lived on the farm for seven years before I asked and Mugwort was not present before my request. I thought it would be safer to ask Mugwort to come than to plant ki, that then the Plant would be less likely to take over. Well, Mugwort arrived within a month. Ki first popped up right next to the door. Then ki started growing in the stone driveway by the barn, then in the disturbed area next to the house (we were still building). By the time I left the farm, four years later, Mugwort had taken over a large area. Therefore, be warned: if you want a clean, tidy garden, Mugwort is not a Plant for you. Or maybe ki is.

There is a belief in folk herbalism that a Plant will appear when ki is needed. I have found this to be true. Some herbalists recommend visiting a client's house to discover who is growing around them and get a sense of what they need. Perhaps, Mugwort is generous because we are in need of ki.

Mugwort is the Plant who made it clear to me that I needed to leave my husband. As I'm writing, I am only now (many years later) realizing that Mugwort began to appear on the farm shortly before helping me to make this life changing decision. Mugwort preemptively surrounded me with support. The Plants assist us in ways that we cannot even imagine.

Plant Spirits

The idea of Plant Spirits may be a new concept to some. Everything that is alive has a Spirit. This Spirit is who animates them and embodies the fullness of this particular Being. Now the question is, who is alive? It is easy for us to understand that humans and animals and even Plants are alive. In truth, all of Nature is alive. This means that Plants, rocks, water, soil, Forests, fish, mushrooms, mountains, and so forth are alive and have a Spirit. We can connect and communicate with this Spirit.

The dominant culture insists that Nature is not alive. Nature is a commodity to be traded, used, and which humans have dominion over. However, Indigenous cultures (those who live as part of Nature) around the world hold a different view. They believe in an animistic world, one where all Beings are alive and Sacred. More and more scientists are discovering that the Indigenous worldview is true. These Beings are not only alive, they are intelligent.

How does our worldview change when we realize that all of Nature is alive and intelligent? Does it make us think twice before cutting a Tree down or poisoning water? Does it make us want to rush out and protect endangered species? Does it make us get down on our knees and look at the ground with wonder? Does it make us want to go to a Forest and listen? I hope so. At least this is what I want to do. Mostly, I hope understanding that Nature is alive and intelligent helps us to remember our place as part of Nature. We are the younger sibling who has much to learn from our more-than-human relatives.

The beauty of working with the Plant Spirits for the healing of our-selves, others, or Nature is that once we create a relationship with them, we always have access. We do not need to ingest anything, which means that we can also work with the Spirits of poisonous Plants. We do not even need to be where the Plants are growing. If we want help, we call on our beloved Plant Spirits, and they remind us that we are never alone and that we are surrounded by unlimited Love and support. The Plant Spirits contain the full matrix of the healing gifts of the Plant we are working with. In other words, we have access to the Whole when we work with the Plant Spirits. In Plant Spirit Healing, the practitioner develops a relationship with a particular Plant, and they then transmit this Plant's Spirit (which some refer to as energy) to their client. The Plant Spirit creates an environment that naturally allows healing to occur, working with the body.

When you consciously communicate with a Plant, you are commu-nicating with the Spirit of that Plant. The Spirit of the Plant is the same for all Plants of that species or variety. For instance, I can connect with a White Ash Tree (*Fraxinus americana*) in Vermont and access the same information and gifts as I can when I connect with a White Ash Tree in Texas. The Spirit of Plants in the same Genus will have similar characteristics. When I connect with a European Ash Tree (*Fraxinus excelsior*) in Ireland, there is a similarity to the White Ash Tree, but the European Ash has other gifts to highlight, specifically helping to regain your sovereignty. I am giving examples with Trees, even though this is Mugwort's chapter, because while the Spirit of the Plant is the same across the species or variety, I have found that some individual Plants have developed their own unique personality. This is particu-larly true with Bushes and Trees who have grown in an area for long periods of time. They adapt to their environment and their experiences of their place help to emphasize certain gifts. This is easily witnessed with Redwood Trees. Sometimes there is a particular Tree or Plant with whom we connect very strongly. Yes, they contain the same Plant Spirit as the other Plants of that species, but there is something special about them. One of my greatest Beloveds is a beautiful Ash Tree who grows at

Sweetwater Sanctuary in Vermont. This Tree has been a major teacher for me. When I need the support of Ash, I call on the Spirit of this particular Ash Tree. In contrast, I do not have a particular individual Mugwort Plant who I am deeply connected with; instead I am connected to the Spirit of the whole species of *Artemisia vulgaris* and this is whom I call on and work with.

Some believe that whenever we work with Plants, we automatically are working with the Spirit of the Plant, which is not true. Working with Plant Spirits is about relationship, intimately knowing a Plant to the point that there is no separation between you. This Plant Spirit lives inside of you. As Pam Montgomery writes, "When one comes to know the spirit of a plant, a merging with the plant takes place and communication freely flows from the plant in the form of insights."[1] I know fantastic herbalists who cannot identify the Plants in the wild. We can make potent herbal medicine without including the Plant Spirit. The medicine can still be effective and our clients can have amazing results. However, we are only working with one component of a Plant. When we work with the Plant Spirit, we have access to the entirety of the Plant's healing gifts and wisdom. To get the most healing, we want to develop a relationship with the Plant Spirit and ask the Spirit of the Plant to be included in our medicine. It is the intention and the relationship that affects the quality of our medicine, which is why it is important to know who is making your medicine or, even better, to make your own.

Plant Spirits have an enormous role in my life, guiding my work, my own healing, and really my life. I want to have a deep, intimate relationship with them. I want to be of service to them. Often, I interchange the words Plants and Plant Spirits because the Plant Spirits are such a large part of my life that there isn't a separation. There are, however, some Plants who are a part of my life and I do not know their Plant Spirit. For instance, I take Rhodiola tincture almost daily. I love Rhodiola, I greatly appreciate ki's healing gifts, and I do not know ki's Plant Spirit. Hopefully that will change one day, but for now this hasn't been necessary nor has the opportunity arisen. It is difficult to be in relationship with a large number of Plant Spirits. If you think about the humans in your life, you may know many, and I'm sure that there are tiers. For example, there are the people you know casually, the people you interact with situationally, the acquaintances you go out with, your work buddies, your family, your support system, and your intimate inner circle. You do not know your acquaintances as well as you know your intimate inner circle. Your inner circle is also smaller than the other groups because time and energy are needed to be able to know one another so well and to maintain your relationships. This is true with Plants and Plant Spirits. I can identify and know the medicinal or edible qualities of a large number of Plants, but am only able to intimately know a relatively small number of Plant Spirits, which is just fine. Thinking that we need to know a large amount of Plant Spirits is amnesia at work. We do not want to consume them, adding another notch. We want to be in deep, conscious relationship with the Plants. These Plant Spirits each have seemingly endless gifts and wisdom to offer us. Therefore we do not need to know hundreds of them.

Anxiety

Mugwort is exceptional at moving and clearing energy. This is why ki is one of the foundational Plants in Plant Spirit Healing. We work with the Spirit of Mugwort for removing stagnant energy, energy blockages, intrusive objects, blocks in the chakras, and more. When a person's energy is chaotic and they are unable to calm or focus, Mugwort works magic. This can occur with anxiety, shock, extreme stress, or trauma. I have had clients who were medicated or even hospitalized for anxiety attacks, and yet they were unable to calm. When they came to see me, their energy bodies were jagged and chaotic;. there was too much energy trapped in their aura, cycling around. I asked Mugwort to help and their energy slowed and started moving downward. They instantly felt calm and could get a sense of themselves again.

Anxiety is incredibly common, though many people continue to be ashamed by their experience of it. My clients with anxiety tend to be sensitive individuals—they sense or feel energies that others do not, and they are often empaths and intuitives. Generally, they also are not grounded, which means they get flooded with energy and information that has nowhere to go. These energies continue to clog their aura and attract more energy and information. The anxiety occurs as their body becomes overwhelmed by these energies and they don't know how to respond or what to respond to. Their nervous system is overloaded.

Since most of this is invisible, other people often do not understand. But when I check my client's aura, I feel like they are surrounded by lightning or fifty televisions all blaring at once. Of course they are struggling. Who could hear themselves or Spirit amongst all that racket?

I have found several things to be helpful in resetting the nervous system and keeping the energies moving: regular energy hygiene, to clear unwanted energies from the aura; daily grounding, to help individuals connect to the Earth and allow these energies to leave on their own (see chapter 5); setting good boundaries, to help reduce the energies coming into one's aura (see chapter 8); and plenty of time in Nature or with animals. Often there are past traumas that need to be healed. Some people developed their sensitive skills as a survival method for avoiding or limiting trauma and abuse. Sometimes they inherited anxiety from their family, learning at a young age to respond to the world in this manner. We may need to work on beliefs and patterns to realign their bodies with safety. Other times we need to look at food sensitivities. Eating foods that they are sensitive or allergic to affects their nervous system (among other things) and contributes to their anxiety. Food sensitivities can create emotional or mental symptoms that get overlooked or discounted. They may also have difficulty releasing or processing toxins. We might need to bring in other supportive methods such as herbs, Flower Essences, baths, exercise, meditation, art. . . . The list is long and depends on the person. If they are open to developing a relationship with Mugwort, ki can be a great support. They can then call on Mugwort anytime they are starting to feel anxious or overwhelmed to help clear their aura and get the energies moving.

While there continues to be a stigma around anxiety, I think it is important to pay attention to those who experience this. They tend to be the canaries in the coal mine, telling us the state of the world. Right now, things are not okay. We are not in alignment with Nature. We are not in alignment with Life. We are hurting each other. We are destroying our Home. There is good reason to be anxious. One could even say that anxiety is the correct response to our situation. That is, unless you listen to Nature. Nature tells us a different story and shows us another way. This is why it is so very important that people who regularly experience anxiety spend as much time as possible in Nature.

Energy Hygiene

We are energetic Beings swimming in a vast sea of energy. As we go through life, we constantly collect and release energy. Some of what we collect is beneficial, but we also absorb what does not belong to us: negative thoughts, fears, emotions, etc. If we do not clear these from our bodies, we attract more of the same. This toxic energy can accumulate and start to wreak havoc on our lives and well-being. Through quantum physics, we understand that we create the world we live in; if our bodies are filled with these negative thought forms and energetic garbage, our world mirrors this. Energy hygiene is the clearing of this "garbage."

Good energy hygiene is vital to our well-being and yet it is something that, in our culture, very few people know about or practice. We recognize the importance of physical hygiene: washing our hair, washing our hands, brushing our teeth, and even eating well and exercising. We understand that these contribute to our health. Through my years of working with clients, I have come to realize that many of our issues, be they physical, emotional, mental, or spiritual, are a result of poor energy hygiene.

Physical illness can arise from accumulated uncleared energy. Energy hygiene is not only essential for good whole-body health, it is also imperative for creating a better world. Carrying around this baggage does not serve anyone. Which means if you are an empath, caregiver, or healer and tend to take on others' problems, then practicing energy hygiene is absolutely necessary for your well-being.

Since Mugwort excels at clearing and moving energy, ki is fabulous for energy hygiene. We smudge with Mugwort to clear the excess and unwanted energies from our energy bodies. Smudging is the act of burning a Plant and using the smoke to affect a person's aura or a space, in this case to clear them. You can do this by creating a smudge stick or simply burning loose leaves.

When we work with the physical Plants, we need to know where they were grown and how they were harvested. Unfortunately overharvesting of medicinal Plants is common, and we can unknowingly contribute to this practice. I recommend referencing the United Plant Savers' Species At-Risk List.[2] With climate change and habitat destruction, this list can change rapidly. As smudging has become more common and mainstream, the need for greater awareness around this practice and the Plants we work with has increased. Many equate smudging with White Sage. White Sage is an At-Risk Plant who is Sacred and important in the ceremonies of many Indigenous communities. We can be respectful relatives by preserving White Sage for the Indigenous cultures to whom ki is Sacred or growing our own.

Fortunately, when there is a need, Nature provides. Get to know your local Plants. Who is good for clearing energy? What Plants did your Ancestors work with? The beauty of Mugwort is that ki grows fast and abundantly, at least where I live. Therefore, Mugwort makes a great resource for smudging. We can, of course, also work with the Plant Spirit for clearing, though sometimes it is nice to have the physical reminder.

To work with a smudge stick, you light the end of it and then gently wave the stick around a person, room, or object, allowing the smoke to remove what needs to be cleared. You can use a large feather or fan to blow the smoke around the person or area you are smudging. It is nice to carry a bowl with you to catch the ashes of the smudge. When you are done, be sure to completely put out the lit end. I stub it out on a shell or heatproof bowl and have a special stone that I use to rub out any other areas that I see are burning (I have had Mugwort smudge sticks burst into fire again because they were not completely extinguished).

To smudge with the dried, loose leaves, place them in a heatproof bowl and light them. Mugwort lights easily. Some Plants or resins may require a charcoal disk or Tinder Polypore for them to remain lit. Holding the bowl in your hand, wave it around the person, room, or object just like you did with the smudge stick (you may want to use a hot pad). When you are finished, you can put out the leaves or allow them to burn until they are finished.

Your intention is important when smudging. I say prayers in my head or audibly, asking the smudge to do what I am wanting. In the case of clearing, I say something (based on a prayer I learned from David Dalton) to the effect of:

"Mugwort, I ask you to clear all densities, low vibrations, stuck or stagnant energies, negative energies, any ill intentions whether conscious or unconscious, intrusive energies, any objects of harm. Please clear my body (or room, etc.) of anything that is blocking my light. Please clear me of negative thought forms, unprocessed emotions, and illness. Please remove these and transmute them. Please infuse my body with light, Love, joy, and healing energy so that I may be in alignment with my Higher Self and the Highest Good of All."

Sometimes it is not appropriate or we do not want to burn Plants (as in an office setting). We can "smudge" with a clearing spray instead. I make mine with 50 percent distilled water and 50 percent vodka as the base. The vodka acts as a preservative and is fairly odorless. To this I add Spirit or Flower Essences who focus on clearing energies and adding protection. I, of course, invite the Spirits of the Plants into this spray. Sometimes I will add essential oils as well, though I often leave the sprays unscented, making it less obvious when they are used. I say the same intention when I spray this on myself and the room.

If you are working with clients, you want to smudge before and after *each* client. I have too many energy workers as clients who only infrequently clear their own energy; this is a prescription for dis-ease on all levels.

A key component to good energy hygiene is being mindful of our thoughts and words. Magic 101 states that whatever you send out, you receive back threefold. When you point your finger, three more are pointing back at you. Lately our dominant culture seems to encourage vitriol and derision under the guise of "telling it like it is" or "speaking one's mind." Hatred and ill-wishes are slung about without consideration of their effects. Words and thoughts carry energy and intention. If we spew hatred, we fill our world and surround ourselves with this energy. We cause harm, even if that is not our intention.

A Shaman we worked with in Ecuador was astonished by the amount of malevolent magic that members of our group carried in their auras, especially since our culture doesn't tend to recognize malevolent magic. Since we don't recognize this possibility, we are not conscious of our thoughts and actions, nor do we regularly participate in energy hygiene and protection. Most of the malevolent magic in our culture may not be intentional, but it still causes great harm, including disease, accidents, and unnecessary drama. We can help reduce these instances while supporting our aura by being conscious of the energies that we add with our words, thoughts, and actions. We can get angry if someone cuts us off in traffic, but we do not need to wish them harm.

It is against Natural Law to interfere with a person's free will, and doing so is a form of malevolent magic. This is obvious when we intentionally cause harm to someone. And it is equally true when our interference has good intentions. When people begin to work with energy healing, they often want to use their new skills to help everyone, including loved ones who have not asked to be helped. Their desire to be helpful hinders their loved ones' free will, thus creating an act of malevolent magic that has negative consequences. It is important to get permission before engaging in energy work and to understand that our actions have energetic impacts. Since Love does not override a person's free will, when in doubt, send Love.

Remembering Our Wild Self

Mugwort, carrying the energy of Artemis, helps us to remember our Wild Self. This is that part of us who never left Nature. For way too long, we have been following a story where humans are separate from Nature. Some even say that humans are in charge of Nature. (Though this last story quickly disappears when a person spends time alone in a truly wild place.) The truth is that we are Nature and Nature is us; there is no separation. We are connected to all Beings. Our bodies are their own ecosystem, containing more bacterial cells than human cells. To say that we have separated from Nature is analogous to saying that we have separated from our right arm (or really our entire body). What we are actually saying is that we have forgotten who we are.

In living with this belief of separation we miss gifts and opportunities, life is more of a struggle than it needs to be, and we need to continually numb ourselves to ignore the loss, as well as the call of something more. For some of us this call is the tiniest whisper that we can barely hear and for others it is a wild roar. That call is coming from the part of us who has not forgotten, our Wild Self.

> *Beloved,*
>
> *It is time to wake. Open your eyes. Receive me into your Heart, your body. Let my blood flow fiercely through your veins again. Remember our connection. Allow your lungs to fill with the exhales of our Green sisters and brothers. Let the Stars decorate your hair. Turn on your Light, remove the shade. Attract your relations. Hoot and holler with ecstasy. Feel the Earth of your body. Allow your Heart to beat to this central rhythm.*
>
> *Let's dance and dance under the Moon, as our skin shimmers with the Silver Light. Let the juices of your body release while we glide to the music that our Hearts hear.*
>
> *I will return, I promise. In truth, I have never left. I've only been waiting for you to remember me, to want me, to yearn for me. I love you. It is soon time.*
>
> *With Love,*
> *Your Wild Self*

As humanity is at a crossroads, it is not surprising to me that Mugwort grows abundantly, asking us to remember. We sacrifice our Integrity to maintain this life of amnesia. We are meant to always do what we said we would, we make vows and promises that we must keep, we work hard and sacrifice, we put others' needs above our own. These are all qualities that are used to describe a person with integrity—a word that is used often and usually as a way of sustaining the dominant paradigm. I, however, use the capital I for Integrity because I am referring to the greatest meaning of this word. We are in Integrity when we are in alignment with our Soul's path. Sometimes in order to be in Integrity, we have to stop being in integrity. In other words, working at a job that makes us sick is not being in Integrity; staying in a toxic relationship, even if we made a vow, is not being in Integrity; ignoring our needs to help someone else is not being in Integrity; saying "yes" when our Soul is screaming "no" is not being in Integrity. The more we choose lowercase integrity, the more we move out of alignment with our Soul. As we do this, our Soul Fire dims and we create energy blockages, making it harder for us to fill up. Mugwort helps to clear these blocks and bring us back into alignment with our Soul and our Integrity. Of course, a big part of Integrity is remembering our connection to All.

If you want to live a path of alignment with Nature, know that Nature is not a fool. Ki requires authenticity and microscopic honesty. We must be honest to our very core, even in our inner thoughts. Our culture encourages deception and suppression. These cause dissonance, resulting in energetic discrepancies and leaks. The other Nature Beings can read these inaccuracies in our auras. Most humans are not this sensitive, but we can notice that we feel uncomfortable around a person who continually lies, even if we just met them. Lies, even white lies, take us out of Integrity; they are a poison that separates us from our wholeness. Nature demands that we own all of ourselves and take responsibility for our actions, both those that help and those that harm. When we stand vulnerable in our honesty, we become trustworthy. We also eliminate the static that surrounds us and reduce the fragmentation of our energy, which allows for a clearer, easier path forward.

The deeper you go, the more authenticity and microscopic honesty is required. This may sound good, even romantic. However, this can be quite brutal and ugly as you are forced to face your hidden aspects and beliefs. It's easy to say that you want to be in Integrity, but are you willing to give up everything that you know to be true? This is a trick question, for as you go about this path, what disappears and ends was not true nor was it in alignment with your Soul. While you can look back at the "difficult" decisions you've made, the truth is you never felt as if you had a choice. For the alternative, living a life where you feel dead inside, never counted as a possibility. I think of the lines from Oriah Mountain Dreamer's poem, "The Invitation": "It doesn't interest me if the story you are telling me is true. I want to know if you can disappoint another to be true to yourself; if you can bear the accusation of betrayal and not betray your own soul; if you can be faithless and therefore trustworthy."[3]

For years, I lived a double life. My then husband and I came to an unspoken understanding: I could do what I wanted during the day, but at night I needed to return to his world and not share my experiences. During the day, I explored with Plants, had many incredible experiences, and learned a lot, but I had to forget these at night. At times, it was hard to live with one foot in each of two worlds, navigating between them. Several months after Yarrow offered to open the doors for me, I experienced a deep grief that left me and my world shattered. As I came back together, I started seeing everything with a different perspective. There were parts of my life that I could no longer accept. By the time I started my Plant Spirit Healing Apprenticeship, I had already started to shift more toward the Plant world. They are the ones who were there for me during my grief. When I stood up for them, they offered me an even deeper experience. As the apprenticeship started, the facade of my relationship began to crumble even more. Following Mugwort into the stream that June day, I unknowingly made a choice: to honor my Wild Self and follow my Soul Path, which also meant leaving my marriage.

From one viewpoint, I removed the keystone of my life. Through this decision, I lost my farm, including the house that my children built;

I lost (and later regained) my relationship with my mother; I lost numerous "friends"; I lost my identity; I left a life of luxury. The worst came a year or so later, when my relationship with my oldest child disintegrated. To this day, this is an enormous pain in my Heart, which brings tears as I write. For as long as I can remember, I wanted to have children. I went through a period of dark depression in high school because I desperately wanted to be a mother and knew that I was too young to raise a child. I was twenty-one when my son was born, so young. And yet he meant everything to me. My whole identity was wrapped up in being a mother. I stayed home with him and, later, his brother. I homeschooled them. When they eventually went to school, I arranged my life so that I could be with them when they were home. Apparently, I needed to learn that I was more than a mother. There are no words to describe how difficult and painful this experience was for me.

Through another viewpoint, I was releasing the parts of me that were untrue. I gained my sense of self. I discovered an incredible support system consisting mostly of amazing, strong, loving, inspiring women who understood my path and believed in me. I let go of a relationship that was killing me and accepted that I had value. I embarked on an unbelievable, magical journey. I started to laugh again.

I now live a life beyond my wildest dreams. Life is no longer a struggle, but a celebration. I said "Yes!" to life and "Yes!" to me. Was it painful? Yes! Would I make the same choice again? Yes! Am I grateful that I left? Every day of my life. And, fortunately, my son and I have a good relationship again. (While I still hurt over that separation, there is a part of me that can admit that it was necessary for both of us.)

Now, this is my story. There are many people who choose to follow their Soul Path and do not need to leave their relationships or jobs. However, I have noticed that the more you cling to something that you think is important (a relationship, a job, a belief, an image of yourself), especially if it demonstrates lowercase integrity, the rockier the dissolution will be. As you go through this process, there may be people who think you are crazy or who try to talk you into maintaining the status quo; in general, we are uncomfortable with change. Another person's change triggers those aspects in our own lives that we are ignoring. What I found is that I was blissfully unaware of this. My path forward was so crystal clear that I did not even hear the detractors. Every day since I made that decision (and probably long before then), the Plants have *always* been there. Any time I struggle on my path, I turn to them. Any time I need guidance, they are there. They have brought such beauty and meaning to my life that the only thing I can do is continue on my path.

Dreaming

My first introduction to Mugwort was as a dreaming herb, which is typical. New herbal students often become enamored with creating dream pillows. Mugwort is amazing at helping us to remember our dreams and tends to make them more vivid. Often there is a warning that Mugwort can create paralyzing nightmares. I have not found this to be true and have asked many people over the years if they have experienced this or know anyone who has and have yet to find confirmation of this warning. One person told me that they did have this happen; however, when I questioned her, she said that she knew she could leave the dream and it was not overly scary. In my experience, if Mugwort brings nightmares, there is a purpose to them, usually letting go of something, confronting fears, or releasing hindrances.

Our dreams were once powerful messengers. We shared them with one another to decipher their meanings and guidance. They were utilized to bring into form what was needed or desired. Many of us have forgotten how to work with our dreams. Some feel that they no longer dream. Mostly this is because we no longer remember our dreams; however, there is research that shows that people who experience depression experience less REM sleep, which is the dream state. If we can remember our dreams, perhaps we can re-member ourselves.

Dreams reveal the truth of our subconscious, showing us areas that we have ignored or that need healing. We process the experiences of our day. We receive deep healing, including bringing back parts of ourselves in our dreams. Robert Moss* writes, "Any dream—even one from thirty years ago—can open the royal road to wholeness and soul recovery."[4] This is a place where we connect with our Soul without our filters or limiting beliefs. Our dreams bring us messages from our Guides or other Beings. Our dreams are portals into other worlds; there is no limit to our dreams. We have access to the wisdom of the universe through our dreams.

Our dreams can lay the groundwork for a situation or experience that we are not quite ready for, preparing us energetically. For instance, I met my past partners in the dreamworld long before I met them in the waking world. I also met the Land that I am currently stewarding in the dreamworld.

As part of Plant communication, we ask a Plant to give us a dream. This dream does not necessarily include the Plant. However, the message or experience of the dream gives an insight into the healing gifts of the Plants. For example, Wendy (who is an excellent dreamer) was getting to know Bleeding Heart. She asked for a dream. That night, she saw huge machinery moving into Sweetwater Sanctuary (where she was studying at the time). The machines were carving up the Land and cutting down the Trees. She didn't understand this dream. Sweetwater is surrounded by Woods that are owned by another organization. Eventually, much later, the machines did arrive. They were there for months, cutting down Trees. The machines left enormous scars on the Land (on all levels). I was there briefly during this time and the Land shook from the machines. It was horrible.

Wendy's dream was prophetic. Even though Bleeding Heart did not appear in the dream, Bleeding Heart was sharing ki's healing gift. Bleeding Heart showed Wendy that ki is an ally and support to help navigate the grief and horror as the Trees were harvested so thoughtlessly. More so, Bleeding Heart can help us when our Hearts are breaking as our world tumbles down around us.

There are many ways that we can receive this information and have these experiences. However, dreaming is free, fairly easy, and we literally do it in our sleep. It feels like an important tool to utilize. Mugwort

---

*Robert Moss has many great books and workshops that can help you strengthen your dreaming skills.

helps us remember how to do this. Ki wants to help encourage us to dream. It is through our dreams that we begin to create the world we want to live in. It is through our dreams that we access the solutions to our issues. It is through our dreams that we re-member who we are. By utilizing this innate tool (and yes, it is innate, even if it is buried), we take ownership of our own experience. No one can interpret your dreams for you. They may give suggestions or point out interesting connections, but your dream is your message. Yes, there are dream dictionaries and there are dream archetypes; however, these are guideposts, not facts. You are the authority of your dreams.

I have found the following list of suggestions to be helpful in improving my ability to remember and learn from dreams:

- Ask Mugwort for assistance. You can ask Mugwort's Plant Spirit or if you prefer a physical connection, drink a cup of Mugwort tea before bed (ki is a bitter) or put a pouch or dream pillow filled with Mugwort inside your pillowcase. (Avoid ingesting Mugwort if you are pregnant.)
- Ask to remember your dreams.
- You can also ask for a dream to help with a certain situation, or ask for a dream from your Plant ally.
- Have a dream journal next to your bed. When you wake from a dream, try to move very little and keep the light off. Sudden movement or noises quickly bring us out of the dream state into the waking state, making it more difficult to remember our dreams. Write down key points from your dream.
- Give your dream a simple descriptive title to help with recalling the dream in the morning. For example, we could title Wendy's dream "Bulldozing Sweetwater."
- Try to get plenty of sleep; if you are rested, it is easier for you to dream and remember your dreams than if you are going to bed completely exhausted.
- If possible, share your dreams with someone soon after waking. Sometimes talking about them helps to trigger a memory.

🍃 Try not to have judgment about your experiences. Judgment is a quick way of erasing meaning and there is no right or wrong way to dream. Remember, dreaming is like a muscle: the more you exercise your dreaming ability, the more comfortable you will be and the easier it becomes.

Imagination

Our dreams are an incredible way of accessing our imagination and one of the culturally acceptable ways of using our imagination. We have to be able to imagine something before we bring it into being. To imagine is to enter the creative process.

Daydreaming and imagining have gotten a bad rap. They are often considered to be lazy activities—or inactivity—by people who are "dreaming" their lives away. However, all great creatives, including amazing scientists, know that they need to take time to let their imaginations wander. It is in these moments where we find the solutions for life's problems or create new innovations.

This ability may seem rusty. Fortunately, the Plants are more than willing to lull us into dreamland, whether we are asleep or wide awake. If you would like to engage with your imagination, Mugwort is a great ally. Ki helps to awaken the inner artist that resides in each of us. Truly, we all are artists. When we stifle or ignore the creative process, we cause an energy blockage in our body. Sometimes this blockage results in dis-ease and sometimes it results in diminished life force energy (which can look like depression). The question is what is your medium or how do you create?

Do you dare to imagine? As I write these words, I hear John Lennon's iconic song. Can we imagine together? And hold the image of this world filled with peace and Love so vividly in our Hearts that we bring this into form?

Moving Toward Wholeness

A number of years ago, Mugwort gifted me a powerful experience. Mugwort was already an enormous Love and ally in my life. Still, ki had plenty of lessons to share with me. During this experience, Mugwort took me out of the dimension in which we currently live into another dimension. From this place, I could see Earth and what was occurring on ki and see experiences from my own life. Mugwort showed me that we live in a paradigm of polarities. We tend to believe in good and bad, though we may disagree which is which. Mugwort helped me to see that in the higher dimensions, the polarities no longer exist and both sides are actually the same. They were both valid and both contributed to the larger energy, just different ways of getting there.

Sometimes I have to work at remembering this experience. It is easy when we are in this current dimension to think that the polarities are real. We can readily become adamant that our way or our beliefs are necessary for the success of Earth or to protect others. We see this now in our political debates. We other those who are not in agreement with us, thus strengthening the polarity. If we could move up to a higher dimension (an ability that Mugwort can gift to us), we would see that these are all false. Humanity is moving in a particular direction. We are evolving. Sometimes the setbacks or the factions we feel are counter to this movement are actually propelling us forward. An example of this is Donald Trump. When he became president of the United States, his words and actions created a large upheaval among its citizens. While one side of the paradigm would say that he has destroyed the environment, destroyed the Constitution, obliterated basic human rights, and so on, if we look at this from another dimension, we see that his actions have also caused more people to focus on their communities. They no longer felt that they could depend on the government; therefore they decided to take action for themselves, protecting Earth, protecting immigrants, protecting women. His actions brought ideas and beliefs that had been hiding and festering into the light so that we could discuss them and heal them. They caused many of us to wake up and become active members of life, working to create the world we have been waiting for.

Even though I am aware of these other dimensions and Mugwort's lessons, I struggle with the polarities demonstrating how strong they are on our Earth. The more we act from them, othering those with different viewpoints, the more we strengthen this paradigm. Therefore, it is important that we try to remember what connects us, what unites us—not just us as humans, but as part of Nature. We all have the same basic needs: healthy food, shelter, clean water, and most importantly Love. When we can feel Love for one another no matter our beliefs, we move into Unity Consciousness and we realize that we truly are all one.

Exercise: Dreaming with Your Plant Ally

- Spend time with your Plant ally.
- Set up your bedroom for good dreaming. If desired, place a dream pillow in your pillowcase. Open your dream journal to an empty page. Place this and something to write with next to your bed. Remove any extraneous light sources.
- As you settle into bed, ask your Plant ally to bring you a dream tonight. Set an intention to remember what you dream.
- Utilize the tips for remembering your dreams: writing down key points, giving titles to your dreams, reducing movement, and discussing your dreams with others.
- In the morning, look over what you wrote or think back over your dreams. Are there any that seem to be connected with your Plant? If so, what is the energy or quality of the dream? Is there a message? Did you receive a healing? Our Plant guides often use the language of symbolism in the dreamworld. Add this information to what you have already gathered from your Plant friend.
- Remember, the dream does not need to include the actual Plant.
- If you can't remember specifics about a dream, ponder how you felt during it. Likewise, if you do not remember a dream, focus on how you felt when you awoke. Those feelings may provide information regarding your Plant ally.
- You can ask for a dream from your Plant as often as needed or desired.

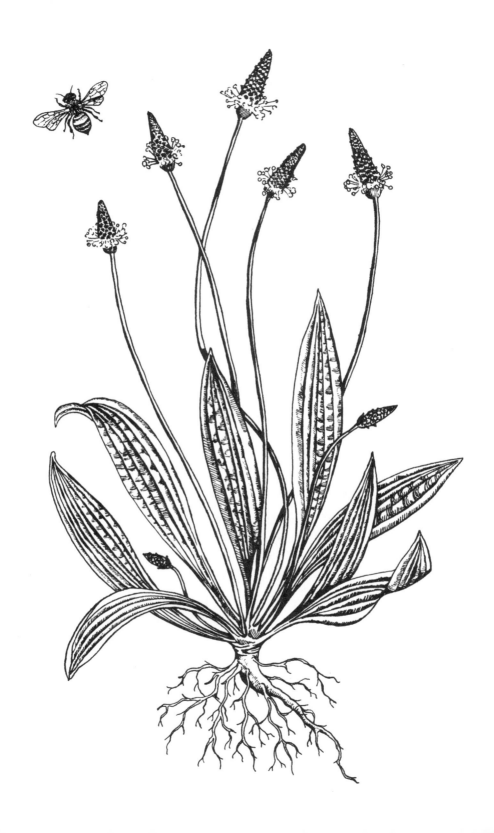

5
❧ Becoming the Authority ❧
Plantain

I often wonder how many favorite Plants I can have. No matter the number, Plantain must be on that list for me. I am referring to the *Plantago* species, not the Plantain that is similar to Banana. The most common species around me are *Plantago major* and *Plantago lanceolata,* though there are over two hundred species worldwide. One of the beauties of Plantain is that they grow everywhere, so wherever I travel, I know that I'll find a friend. I even found one growing in the caldera at Volcano National Park!

Plantain is a rather unassuming Plant. Most people do not even know that ki exists; they simply think ki is part of the Grass. Or they may know Plantain as that "weed" who is destroying their perfect lawn. Yet Plantain continues, quietly waiting for you to realize how wonderful and, in Plantain's own words, powerful ki is.

I always include Plantain in an herb walk. People often respond, "But this grows in my backyard!" Yes, yes, ki does and that is the point. You have invaluable medicine growing right outside your door. This medicine can help you in emergency situations as well as help you maintain your health.

Introducing Children to Plants

Plantain excels at drawing out toxins. This is one of the main reasons why ki is usually the first Plant that I share with children. Children naturally want to experience their environment, especially Nature. Unfortunately, their innate love of Nature can be stymied by the fears and opinions of the adults in their lives. (And, of course, by any trauma that the children have experienced.) A common fear for children (and adults) is being stung by bees. Bees are amazing Beings. Much of our food is dependent on bees pollinating the Plants. And then, there's honey—who doesn't love honey? Well, my mom doesn't, but still, honey is such a wondrous and delicious gift, as well as an incredible medicine, created by the bees. I can spend hours watching bees dance from flower to flower gathering pollen. I enjoy capturing pictures of their butts hanging out of flowers, though I don't succeed at this often; they seem to be a little shy about having their behinds photographed.

The fear of being stung can far outweigh the incredibleness of bees and can greatly inhibit one's enjoyment of Nature. Some people have severe allergic reactions to bee stings and anaphylactic shock is serious. Still, I know people who are allergic to bee stings and continue to be enamored of these amazing Beings. They don't let this life-threatening condition stop them from experiencing Nature, though it might be advisable to keep an EpiPen nearby.

What does Plantain have to do with appreciating bees? Ki is an incredible remedy for bee stings, helping to pull out the toxins and thus reducing the pain, swelling, and heat, sometimes instantly.

I want to empower children (and adults) to explore the wonders of Nature. Giving them tools for reducing their fears or risks of being hurt allows them to be more courageous in their explorations. Besides, Plantain is a fantastic kid-friendly ambassador to the Plant world. In order to work with Plantain for a bee sting, the child chews up a leaf and spits this out onto the sting, creating a poultice. Someone else can do this, but it is best if the person who was stung chews up the Plantain leaf. Remove the poultice when it becomes warm and replace with a new one, repeating until the pain and swelling disappears. Wasps' stings are alkaline and therefore it is helpful to first neutralize the sting with vinegar. Plantain poultices can still help, but are usually less effective without vinegar.

Many years ago, we had a gathering at our farm. One of my children's friends would break down whenever he felt pain or was bleeding. Of course, he got stung at our gathering. He immediately started screaming, "I'm dying! I'm dying!" I quickly grabbed a Plantain leaf, had him chew it, and put it on the sting. He stopped crying, calmed down, and looked at me in amazement with his big, beautiful eyes. We did this a few more times, then he forgot about the sting and went and played with the other kids.

Once a child experiences the incredible healing of Plantain (or another Plant), they want more. They look at Nature with new eyes, seeing that they are supported and loved. They want to know what other Plants can be eaten or can help their injuries. The world becomes a safer place. Isn't that what we want for our children—for them to feel safe and loved?

Of course, Plantain is beneficial for adults as well. Ki is an incredible Plant for drawing out toxins, including snake venom, splinters, shards of glass, debris from wounds, lung irritants, and infections such as infections of the mouth, lung, intestines, and more. If you are going to do any hiking or back country exploration, Plantain is a great Plant to know. There are many stories shared about Plantain saving people's lives until they could receive medical care. Plantain has many healing gifts.

Plants as Rebellion

Knowing how to heal ourselves and how to make our own medicines is a subversive act in a capitalist society. It also is one of the fundamental skills of our Ancestors. It is helpful to work with healers as they can usually see a broader picture of us than we can and hopefully they have more training than we do. However, everyone should know basic home health care, such as what to do for a bee sting, how to treat a cold or the flu, what to do with a fever. Not only is this often cheaper and more effective, it also is a way of reclaiming authority for our lives.

In a capitalistic, patriarchal culture, wealth is created by convincing you that you do not know how to take care of your body. You need their product. You need to buy their advice. Or even that your body is wrong: wrong shape, wrong size, wrong color. This continues in our current "healthcare" system—in quotes because it is not clear to me that this system is focused on health; it seems to be focused on creating long term clients and then focusing on disease, which is the opposite of health.

I have clients with long lists of diagnoses who have been working with the allopathic system for years while their symptoms continue to worsen. They went to countless doctors before anyone believed that they were experiencing pain. If the doctors weren't able to find an explanation for their pain on a diagnostic test, they were told that there isn't anything physically wrong, that it must be psychological and, often, they were given antidepressants. Other times they were treated as if they were addicts looking for pain medication. None of this helped their situation. Sometimes there was a good physical explanation for their experience, such as Lyme disease, but the doctors did not recognize it nor did they order the correct diagnostic tests. Other times, their pain or symptoms were their body's way of getting their attention, to urge them to heal their trauma or emotional wounds, which is different from diagnosing their issue as psychological. Saying a person's experience is psychological is saying that they are making it up, they are creating their pain or symptoms for a reason. Recognizing that the pain is being caused by their trauma or emotional wounds accepts that the pain is real and has a purpose. Even more importantly, when we understand that purpose, we can create a shift so that it is no longer needed.

Please understand I am not criticizing doctors, but the system in which they must participate. I have clients who are doctors, and they've shared with me the terrible challenges of only being able to spend a short amount of time with each patient and the large number of patients they see every day, which means that they are unable to fully listen and focus on each person. In addition, their training cannot cover everything that a body can experience or all that can help a body come back into alignment with health. If a person does not present with very clear symptoms that fit nicely into a diagnostic box, then they might be ignored or their symptoms may be discounted.

It can be tempting to hand control of our bodies and our health to someone else. However, no one else can understand our body better than we can. We are the ones who inhabit this body every minute of our life. Only we know how the sensations feel or how our body reacts. Sometimes we need help in understanding these sensations or even recognizing them. Sometimes we need a guide to encourage us to continue through our healing journey or to remind us of who we truly are. But in the end, only we can be responsible for our health and our body. Not taking ownership of our health and experiences creates an energy leak.

Plants encourage us to increase our awareness of our body and how we interact with the world. They help to bring us into the present moment and become conscious of our senses and experiences. They help us to stand in our center and know: know what we should eat, know what is right for us, know what decision to make . . . ultimately, they help us know who we are.

When we have this understanding, it doesn't matter what anyone else says or thinks, for we know the Truth. We can then stop giving our power away to others and can utilize this energy for sharing our unique gifts with the world.

Becoming the Author(ity) of Your Life

As I've emphasized, the Plants meet us where we are and provide the information that we most need at that time. We can continue to learn from the same Plants for our entire lives. If you are communicating with a Plant, they may give you information or tell you how to work with them in a way that is very different from an herb book or what someone else would suggest. This is wonderful! The Plant just gave you an incredible gift. You would not want to show disrespect by ignoring that information because someone else did not have that same experience. (Although, of course, we may want to use discernment regarding the information that we have received.)

The more we listen to the Plants and the more we trust our own experience, the more we become the authority of our life. Aren't we the best person for this role? Certainly, we are a better authority than a magazine or talk show host or business. The beauty is that as we become the authority, we also become the author of our life. We are all handed situations and opportunities, and it is up to us to decide how these will affect us and what we will do with them. When we are unsure, over-whelmed, or confused, it is helpful to go to the Plants to gain a differ-ent perspective.

As the author of my life, I consider the Plants to be my muse. They make suggestions, helping me to decide what I shall create. Sometimes these suggestions save me or help me to make a better choice than I would have on my own.

When we first moved onto the farm, only three Plants grew there: Burdock, Thistle, and Jimsonweed. We asked a local farmer to plant Hay to help keep the soil covered until we had a better plan for what the farm wanted. My neighbor had an enormous area that was filled with Plantain and yet no Plantain would grow at the farm. It took me years to coax Plantain to grow just a few feet away. In time, we also had patches of Plantain.

Plantain is sometimes referred to as White Man's Footprint because of ki's tendency to grow where the European colonists lived and moved. Plantain likes to grow near people in disturbed, compacted ground. It was unusual that it took so long for Plantain to appear on the farm. But because of this, I was very aware of ki's growing spots. With two active children, we relied heavily on Plantain for bee stings, insect bites, and removing splinters or other tiny irritants.

My oldest son cut his thumb and required stitches. (I did not have access to Yarrow at the time.) Unfortunately, the doctor did a poor job and his thumb became infected. It was red, hot, and swollen; I was concerned about a possible blood infection. I went to harvest Plantain to help draw out the infection. I always ask permission before harvest-ing and let the Plants know why I would like to harvest them. I said my prayers and went to a large Plantain spot, only there wasn't any

Plantain. Red Clover was there instead. I greeted Red Clover and asked ki to help me find Plantain. I went to another one of Plantain's usual spots and had the same experience. I thanked Red Clover and said, I really need Plantain, please help me. I went to a third Plantain spot and again there was no Plantain, but Red Clover was shining. Finally, I realized that Red Clover helps with infections, especially blood infections. I thanked both Plantain and Red Clover, harvested Red Clover, and made a strong tea to soak my son's thumb in. The infection cleared and I understood that Plantain and Red Clover were showing me who was the best remedy for my son at that time. I greatly appreciate the extreme patience of the Plant Beings; sometimes we humans can be a little slow to understand, yet they keep showing up and guiding us until we are ready to learn.

We live in an amazing, beautiful world. The more I spend time with and study Nature, the more I believe in magic and infinite possibilities. Whatever the need, Nature provides the solution (if we are willing to ask and listen). I have a shirt that says, "There's a Plant for that." It's true. Often the Plants show up with their healing gifts before we even realize that we need them. I think of this with Plantain and how ki followed Europeans around the world as we colonized, raped, and destroyed the peoples, cultures, and Lands we encountered. Plantain patiently followed with a remedy waiting for us to recognize the need.

Transmuting the Trauma of Colonialism

For too long the wounds of colonialism, white supremacy, and patriarchy have been festering. These systems are toxins that poison and destroy life. Schools and history books teach that this is history, as in something that occurred a long time ago for which we are not responsible and about which we can do nothing. It takes very little effort to see that these systems continue today, as evidenced by police officers kneeling on the necks of Black men, oil pipelines being routed through Native American Sacred sites and water supplies, mass incarceration rates for Black and Native American people, high sexual assault and rape rates of women, the murdered and missing Indigenous Women, the gender pay gap, voter restriction laws, multinational corporations destroying the Amazon Rainforest for oil and beef; the list goes on and on.

The point is that colonialism, white supremacy, and patriarchy are alive and continue today. The wounds are fresh. It does not matter who your Ancestors are or what they did or didn't do, you are affected by this and there is healing work to be done. There are many different reactions to this—some want to dive in and focus on the healing 24/7, looking at every possible thread, while some are overwhelmed by the pain and need to grieve; some may take on the guilt of every act, while others deny that these systems continue, deny their impact, or respond with anger. The truth is that these responses are all part of the healing process. Anyone who has done personal healing work knows that anger and denial are definite stages along the way, even for those who are most dedicated to Love and healing. What we need when we are experiencing these is compassion. We need to be held in Love, for our wounds, fears, and limiting beliefs are being activated.

Shame and blame do not have a role in healing. We need to acknowledge the wounds and impacts of these systems and realize that we are all accountable for shifting and healing them, especially those who profit from them. Leah Penniman states, "One of the highest forms of love is accountability."[1] Our fear can take over when we think about shifting these systems, for we have a sense of the pain that is involved. It can be painful when we begin to look at the roots and impacts of these systems; however, we often discover that shifting them is liberating, for we have been unknowingly carrying that pain around with us. We all benefit from the healing. Sometimes I think the people who have seemingly profited from colonialism, white supremacy, and patriarchy have the most to gain from the healing of these systems, for their Souls, our Souls, are hurting.

Plantain can help those who are ready to actively engage in the healing of these systems. Working with the Plant Spirit of Plantain helps to clear your energetic system of the imprints of colonialism. We also work with Plantain to clear the energetic imprints that are held in the Land. I live in an area where there were massacres of the Conestoga Indians. The energy from these atrocities remains. I can feel it when I walk into certain areas. The Land (and often the Trees) holds the trauma for us because it is too great for humans to handle. However, in order for there to be healing, the trauma needs to be transmuted. Plantain is one of the Plants who can help us with this, removing the toxins of the trauma from the Land.

This does not excuse us from doing the work of changing the systems. It is humans who created this mess and humans who need to be engaged in the healing and shifting. However, since most of us are amnesiacs and cannot even imagine a world where these systems aren't the basis of our culture, the Plants are here to help guide us through the healing and creating of a world that is aligned with Life, where all Beings are treated as Sacred.

Clearing Toxic Emotions

Sitting with Plantain, I feel a drawing motion, pulling toxins out of my body and transmuting them into white light. My spine becomes a beam of white light as my body is being cleared of toxic emotions.

We can engage with Plantain's incredible drawing capacity to clear out the held emotions that are poisoning us. Many of us were taught that there are good emotions and bad emotions. We want to express the good emotions (happiness, contentment, joy) and are often rewarded when we do. If we express the bad emotions (anger, jealousy, grief) then something is wrong with us, or we might be punished. This is simplified, but I think you know what I'm talking about. This myth of good and bad emotions is shared even in the natural healing field.

Let's be clear, there is no such thing as a good or bad emotion. All emotions have a role. It isn't the emotion that is problematic but what we do with that emotion or how we respond. Emotions are meant to help us experience the sensations of life on Earth. They help us know that we are alive; they enliven and clear our energetic system. They are signposts along our path, helping us decipher our experiences. We are meant to feel them, learn what they are telling us, and release them, which then clears the space for the next lesson and emotion.

When we suppress or ignore an emotion, we ignore the wisdom of our bodies. Sometimes we do this until we no longer know what we are feeling. Other times, we react inappropriately to situations because they trigger these held emotions. Rejecting or suppressing an emotion creates stagnation, which becomes a magnet gathering more and more emotions. Like any blockage, suppressing emotions creates an imbalance in our body, leading to dis-ease and pain. It does not matter what the emotion is—we poison ourselves when we stifle it.

I recently experienced more than a year of very intense intestinal issues including debilitating pain. During my healing process, I discovered trapped emotions. It was amazing to see these emotions come up. When they did, I got curious about what was beneath them and discovered that some connected to experiences going as far back as elementary and middle school. It was liberating to feel these emotions; I was tapping into my full potential and felt powerful and alive.

We are meant to experience all of our emotions. Ideally, we can notice and name them. I like to pause throughout the day and ask myself what I am feeling. I often refer to a feelings chart to help me clarify what I am feeling, broaden my awareness of possible emotions, as well as understand what is not a feeling or emotion. The Center for Nonviolent Communication has a nice list of feelings that I often suggest for my clients.[2]

Then we get curious: "Why am I feeling this? What is behind this emotion?" Sometimes we discover that we are reacting to something from our childhood or a past relationship. Sometimes it is because someone is treating us inappropriately, or because a need isn't getting met. Sometimes we are experiencing a beautiful moment and are feeling seen and loved.

Then we decide how to respond. Perhaps we say, "Please do not speak to me that way." Perhaps we spend time in Nature restoring ourselves. Perhaps we let our tears flow. Perhaps we do healing work to clear the previous trauma. Remember, if we are experiencing held emotions, we can ask Plantain to draw them out and transmute them. Plantain helps to clear the toxicity from these poisons.

While we do want to feel and express our emotions, we do not want to be ruled or consumed by them, reacting like a ping pong ball, bouncing from one extreme to another as we respond to our experiences. Babies are a great example of this. They quickly go from happy as can be to full out screaming to snuggling and sucking their thumb within thirty seconds. That is appropriate for a baby—it is how they communicate with their loved ones. But as adults, we have more skills available. It is exhausting (to you and everyone around you) to go from one extreme to another. Ideally, we feel our emotions from a grounded state, so that we can notice, get curious, and express ourselves, all while staying centered in our Being. Fortunately, Plantain helps us to center and ground.

Grounding

Plantain is a fairly small Plant who often appears to be part of the soil. The seedhead can be quite long and generally stands very straight, almost like a miniature Mullein Plant. When I sat with Plantain, I felt my body sinking into the Earth and my spine aligning. I could feel myself connected to the Earth below and the sky above, a conduit of energy and information. From this place I could feel my connection to everything and my unique place in this world. The worries drained from me as the Earth received and transmuted them. They were replaced with a sense of calm and an increased flow of energy. Plantain helped me to ground.

Grounding is an incredible technique that brings us into the present moment and calms and centers us. Grounding helps us to remember our connection to all and helps to energize us. I frequently suggest grounding techniques for my clients. Grounding is simple and yet has great effects.

We have a tendency to avoid staying in our bodies; we dissociate, we don't want to feel what we feel, or we want to transcend our physical experience. We also tend not to be in the present moment, either fixating on what has already occurred or worrying about what might occur in the future. All of this keeps us from fully experiencing our life and this incredible world, from really appreciating the gifts and beauty that surround us. Grounding helps to change this. Like any skill, the more we do this, the easier it becomes to quickly move into an embodied, present awareness.

If we are struggling with being grounded, focusing first on being in our Heart center can help. We may also need to heal trauma, since trauma can disrupt our ability to feel safe, embodied, and connected. We can call on Plants to help us ground. Trees are natural supports for grounding as they have incredible roots and their trunk and branches are physical manifestations of the energy flow. Of course, Plantain is a powerful ally for helping us to ground and connect with Earth.

A Note

Hopefully it is clear that Plantain helps to draw or pull out something whether it is a splinter, a bee sting, a held emotion, or the wounds of colonialism. This is Plantain's incredible healing gift. It is important to be aware if you are going to work with Plantain that ki can also bring up the aspects of ourselves that we generally try to avoid. These can be the parts of ourselves that are not considered pretty or appropriate in our culture. Generally, these aspects are connected to our Soul's lessons, our wounds, and our healing work. There truly is nothing wrong with them. However, it is possible that if Plantain begins to bring them up, you may feel uncomfortable or may not want to experience them—although sometimes we need to experience a little discomfort to bring forward freedom. Please understand that Plantain is doing so only to help you embrace your wholeness and gifts. Trying to suppress or conquer them perpetuates a warring mentality. They are a part of us. Rather than suppress or conquer, we need to embrace and love. We hold these hidden parts in compassion and understanding and listen to the wounded aspects of ourselves. When we notice the wounded parts arising (for example, we feel jealousy), we get curious, we give voice to them, we listen, we become the parent comforting the hurt child. What needs aren't being met? What wants healing? What beliefs are popping up? If it feels like too much, you can ask Plantain or another ally for support.

Exercise: *Grounding with Your Plant Ally*

Grounding is a practice that is beneficial to us and can help us to connect with our Plant ally.

- If you can, it is nice to do this exercise outside with your Plant friend, but if that's not possible, invite the Spirit of your Plant ally inside.
- My preference is to do this while standing. You can also modify this for sitting or even laying down.
- If standing, you want your feet about shoulder width apart, knees slightly bent. If seated or lying down, make yourself comfortable, being sure that you feel supported by the ground or other surface beneath you.
- You may want to move your body around, shaking out any tension.
- Close your eyes and take several deep breaths, relaxing your body. If you have any areas of tension, direct your breath to them. Take a deep breath again, feel your body expand with your breath, sensing the edges of your body. If you need to, you may shift your body or move your feet to find a comfortable position.
- When you are ready, on your next exhale allow yourself to feel your roots stirring at the base of your spine and the bottoms of your feet. Feel free to use your imagination to visualize your roots.
- With the next exhale, these roots begin to grow. If you are inside, they go through the floorboards and through any other floors necessary to reach the Earth. If outside, they enter the ground.
- With each exhale, your roots grow fast and strong. They mingle with the roots of your Plant ally. Feel this connection. Remember that you can exchange information and energy through these roots.
- Now with your next exhale, your roots go deeper, growing around the bones of the Ancestors, the Ancestors of the Land you are standing on as well as the bones of your own Ancestors. Feel the support.
- Growing deeper still, your roots travel through the layers of stone, through the very bedrock.
- Exhaling again, your roots tap into the underground aquifers, absorbing the wisdom of these ancient seas. Your roots continue growing deeper and deeper.

- Your roots grow all the way down to the very center of the Earth, to the molten lava.

- Spend some time here feeling the energy of the Earth, feeling your connection to the very center. Sense the power and wisdom of this vast energy source.

- When you are ready, use your inhalation to begin to draw this energy up through your roots, like a great straw. Know that you have the ability to control the flow of energy you draw up: increasing the flow if you need more energy or decreasing the amount if it is too much for you. As you suck this energy up through your roots, you create a lovely symbiotic exchange of nourishment, wisdom, and connection among all the Beings who come in contact with it.

- Draw the energy from the center of the Earth up your roots, bringing it higher and higher, the energy flowing faster than you can imagine.

- Bring the energy up through the aquifer.

- Draw it up through the bedrock and the other stone Beings.

- Bring it past the bones of the Ancestors.

- Bring the energy up to where your roots are connected with your Plant ally's roots, sharing the energy with your Plant.

- Bring the energy up through the ground or the floor, all the way up to the bottoms of your feet and to the base of your spine. Allow this energy to feed and balance your root chakra, helping you to feel safe and connected.

- Draw this energy up from the center of the Earth and bringing it into your second chakra, the area between your pelvis and your belly button, helping you to be receptive, creative, and aligned with pleasure.

- As you inhale, bring this energy up to your solar plexus or third chakra, the area just above your belly button. Feed and balance this chakra, helping you to shine your unique star, sharing your gifts with the world.

- Draw the energy up into your Heart chakra. Fill this chakra with the Earth's energy, helping you receive and give Love, helping you to be Love.

- Bring that energy up to your throat chakra, helping you to express your Truth.

🍂 Draw that energy up to your first eye chakra, the place just above the brow line in the center of your forehead. Feed this chakra, helping you to gnow (know intuitively) and to see clearly.

🍂 Draw the energy all the way from the center of the Earth to your crown chakra, at the top of your head, helping you to remember that you are connected to the Divine, that you are a Divine Being incarnated.

🍂 Allow your crown chakra to open like a flower, as the energy from the center of the Earth flows through your chakras and out of the crown chakra, rising higher and higher, into the center of the sky.

🍂 This beam of energy continues to grow higher and higher with each inhale, until the beam is surrounded by star dust.

🍂 This beam continues to grow, reaching your special star. Pause here. You are connected to the center of the Earth, your Plant ally, and your special star. You are connected to all. Through this beam you are able to receive energy, information, nourishment, and healing. Feel the connection.

🍂 When you are ready, allow the beam to branch down like a great Willow Tree, bringing energy from your star back to the Earth, completing the cycle of giving and receiving.

🍂 Open your eyes. If you like, you can give any excess energy that remains in your body back to the Earth by placing your hands on the Earth or the floor, giving gratitude for the generosity of Earth and your Plant Being.

🍂 Notice how you feel.

🍂 Spend time with your Plant ally, listening and connecting.

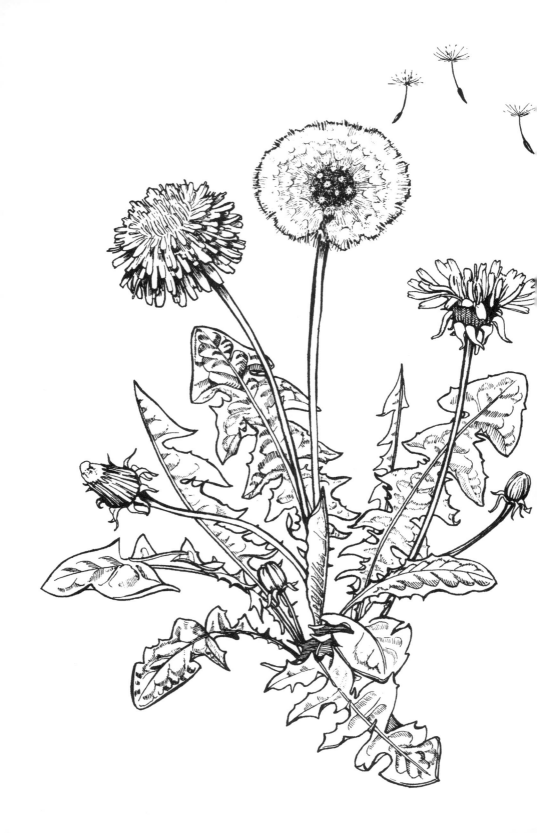

6
❧ Resiliency ❧
Dandelion

*I*f there is a Plant who begs to be met with innocent perception, ki is Dandelion, the beloved Plant of children and herbalists and the dreaded weed of lovers of the green lawn and immaculate gardens. Like Plantain, Dandelion is not native to the United States. Dandelion also arrived here with the colonial settlers, though they intentionally brought Dandelion with them because of ki's medicinal and edible qualities. Dandelion is exceedingly common, making it easy to overlook ki or to think that we know all that there is to know about Dandelion. Spend time with Dandelion and you will quickly discover that there is much to learn, for ki is a generous Plant with many gifts.

Dandelion is the first Plant that I worked with in my Plant Spirit Healing Apprenticeship. I remember seeing Birch waving to me across the creek. When I went to ki, I didn't feel a connection but I looked down and saw Dandelion shining brightly. Dandelion was the perfect Plant for me at that time. My sense of self and my self-esteem were completely shattered, and ki assisted me in remembering who I was in my core. Ki helped me to be comfortable in my body and to love myself again. Dandelion brought the pieces of me back together so that I could follow my path, for I would need the confidence, self-Love, and strength to leave my marriage.

Tenacity and Resilience

Several years ago, Rosemary Gladstar spoke at the MidAtlantic Women's Herbal Conference. As she talked about Dandelion, she giggled in her Rosemary way, commenting on a weed killing company using Dandelion as part of their logo. She said, "It's ridiculous because Dandelion is winning." Which is absolutely true. Dandelion is the embodiment of tenacity. Dandelion grows where Dandelion wants to grow: in the middle of the street, in cracks in the sidewalk, in the garden . . . all the poisons that are spread do not kill Dandelion. Ki will come back again. Pull Dandelion out and ki will return. Mow Dandelion and ki will develop a shorter stalk. Dandelion says, "Hit me with your best shot. You won't kill me. I will continue to sit here shining for all to see while I feed the bees."

I think we can use some of that kick-ass Dandelion-ness, being confident in who we are and thriving wherever we are planted. Fortunately, Dandelion is willing to help us. The yellow blossom is practically a signature for the third chakra. This is the area that is located between your belly button and Heart, the place of your unique star. The third chakra helps us to know ourselves and to share our authentic self with the world. For those who are not confident or are afraid of being seen, Dandelion helps you shine your light brightly. Like Dandelion, when we know ourselves, nothing can destroy us. We might get knocked down or perhaps need a break, but we will return shining brightly, for that is what we are meant to do: shine.

If we are struggling and feeling beaten by the world, Dandelion can help us remember our inner resources. Ki is a survivor who encourages us to find our roots and thrive. Thriving requires resiliency and adaptability while remaining centered. Dandelion growing through the cracked asphalt is the embodiment of thriving. Dandelion tells us, "No matter which way the wind blows you, always find your roots." Finding your roots is both grounding or connecting with Earth and knowing who you are in the core of your Being. Dandelion can assist you if you need help with this.

As we navigate our quickly changing world and the astonishing amount of toxins that surround us, Dandelion's guidance is invaluable. Dandelion root supports our livers and helps them to remove toxins from our body. Dandelion Plant Spirit helps us release the emotional, psychological, and energetic toxins we have accumulated, including those connected to past traumas. When we remember that Plants appear where they are needed, it is no wonder that we find Dandelion everywhere. We also can see the absurdity in spreading poisons in an attempt to eradicate the very remedy to those poisons.

Authentic Experience

Spending time with Dandelion brings forth childlike playfulness. The bright yellow flowers engender joy, especially as they are some of the earliest Plants to blossom in the Northeast. Sometimes Dandelion will even bloom during winter, an exceptionally joyful sight. And then the seedheads, well, they beg you to blow them or dance with them and remember the joy and innocence of childhood. This seemingly innocent, playful Plant is a powerful healer.

While Dandelion does elicit joy, ki also brings up anger. This experience can be surprising to people who are beginning their journey with Plants. There is a preconceived notion that working with Plants is light, joyful, and airy-fairy, which is only partially true. The Plants help us to have an authentic experience of life, feeling the painful and the pleasurable, for both are essential.

I have had students use unpleasant experiences with Plants to validate their stories that something is wrong with them. I ask them to share the information that they received, including the sensations they were feeling and the stories that were playing in their head. Often, the Plants are demonstrating their healing gifts or are helping the student to become aware of a wound. When we have an unpleasant experience with a Plant, we may want to run away. If we can stay and sit with the pain, the Plants will guide us toward a resolution. Ultimately, this reduces the pain and trauma we have been carrying, helping us to feel more whole.

Do not underestimate the power of Plants. We may think that they are sweet and gentle, and they can be, but if you get to know them you will find yourself on your knees crying, sometimes in awe and gratitude, sometimes in release or acknowledgment of pain. You never quite know where your journey will lead.

The Sacred Role of Anger

Anger is one of the emotions categorized as "bad," but it has a very important role to play. Mahatma Gandhi told his grandson, Arun Gandhi, "Anger to people is like gas to the automobile—it fuels you to move forward and get to a better place. Without it, we would not be motivated to rise to a challenge. It is an energy that compels us to define what is just and unjust."[1]

Anger lets us know when our boundaries have been crossed and, if we can direct it appropriately, we can quickly repair those boundaries. For example, if someone calls us a degrading name, we can respond, "Please don't call me that." We don't have to yell or smash something; we simply set a boundary. Other times anger requires action. For instance, when a police officer kills an unarmed Black person, there are protests in the streets, or we write letters and make phone calls to our legislators. We need to do something. Our anger helps us to discern this act as unjust and against Life.

There is much in this world that is unjust. The basis of our society is out of alignment with Nature and Life. When we engage in anger too much, we run the risk of burning ourselves out, or becoming consumed by righteous anger, which serves no one. We want to utilize our anger in healthy ways to create a more just and equitable world. As with every emotion, we need balance, which begins by recognizing the role of anger.

The belief that anger depletes the immune system surfaces from time to time in different circles. This belief denies anger's validity, however, and helps to support the understanding that anger is bad and that we must always be going forward, always growing, always improving, and always at peak performance.

I find it ironic that I am writing about anger, because I have been afraid of anger for most of my life. And yet this is what happens when we work with the Plants—they recognize our challenges and wounds and help us to heal. I once participated in a Dandelion ceremony. I had great expectations, thinking it was going to be a blissful, out of this world experience. However, the number one rule is to not have expectations. Sure enough, as the ceremony progressed, I felt anger building and building. I wrote in my notes, "I feel Dandelion bringing up anger and irritation." Many years later, Dandelion continues to teach me about anger.

What I thought was anger when I was younger was actually rage. This was anger that built up until it exploded, projected toward someone for some small occurrence. The screaming, seething, spitting faces we see in the news are not faces of anger, but faces of trauma and fear turned into rage. When we are unable to feel and express all of our emotions, often anger or rage become the masks that we wear to prevent ourselves from noticing the pain below the surface. It is helpful if we can remember this. When anger starts to surface for us, we can get curious to see if this is appropriate. Has a boundary been crossed? Has a wound been touched? Are we trying to deflect? When someone else is directing anger at us that doesn't feel justified, if we are brave, we can meet their anger with Love and curiosity, recognizing that most likely they are expressing their trauma. There is a beautiful podcast with Ruby Sales where she suggests asking the question, "Where does it hurt?"[2]

During my healing journey, I discovered a large amount of repressed anger that had left my digestive system in shambles. While it may be true that anger depletes the immune system for a number of hours, that is nothing compared to what occurs when we repress our anger. Repressing our anger sets us up for long term dis-ease and disconnection from our bodies.

As I sorted through my repressed anger, I revisited situations that occurred in middle school, high school, and earlier. I was reminded of horrible, completely inappropriate things that the boys in my school said to me. I generally ignored them and kept smiling. Looking back, I see that I internalized their attacks. Rather than confronting their bad behavior, I took these comments to mean that something was wrong with me. I started dimming my light. This ultimately led me to not feel worthy of Love and settling for relationships with people who were abusive toward me. I understand that the boys were simply trying to find their own way in the world and were acting out the roles they thought they were supposed to play. I wonder how much more pain I contributed to because I didn't meet these attacks with anger and boundaries. Perhaps if I had spoken up, the boys would have learned how to respectfully treat other people. Perhaps it would have even kept someone from being sexually assaulted. I have no way of knowing, but I do know that repressing the anger created a poison inside me and kept me from truly sharing my gifts in this world.

The liver and gallbladder are the organs associated with anger. Since Dandelion supports both of these organs, it is no surprise that Dandelion helps bring forward repressed anger. Anger is simply an emotion, a notification that something is going on. The question is, how do we respond to this notification?

Again, I like to be curious when I experience an emotion. Sometimes with anger it is very clear—that man rubbed up against me, let's create a boundary and let him (and others) know that this is inappropriate. Other times the root of the anger is not obvious. Anger likes movement; really, anger requires movement. I tend to go for a walk in order to start processing. I ask myself, is there an action or experience that I am angry about? What about this elicits anger? Does this remind me of something in my past? Is my feeling appropriate? Is there something else? Perhaps I have a need that isn't being met. Perhaps I haven't been taking time for myself and my resources (and tolerance) are running thin. Is there something that needs to occur or shift?

Fire is amazing. Ki is cleansing, life giving, and destructive. There is a big difference between a campfire or a controlled burn used to rejuvenate the Land and an enormous Forest fire raging out of control, destroying anything and everything in ki's path. If we want to be in alignment with Nature then we want our anger to be expressed like a controlled burn, directed only toward those who are involved, allowing the anger to rejuvenate and helping the dormant seeds of beauty to sprout. When we do not do our personal work or investigate the anger, our anger can easily become rage, burning indiscriminately.

Anger can be an incredibly effective tool when we are healing our traumas. People who have been abused can imagine themselves in a particular scene and utilize their anger to fight back, say "No!" or tell the abuser what they think of them. It may be helpful to do this in a safe, therapeutic situation with someone who can guide you through the process and who is comfortable being around large emotions. Sometimes we just need to scream. This helps us to get in touch with our primal selves. It is helpful to do this where you feel safe and unselfconscious, because we want to bear down and really roar, connecting with your "Wild Animal," as my teacher Rocío Alarcón, would say. It is amazing how cathartic this can be. Sometimes we need to break something. I know someone who bought used dishes and smashed them in their garage. This helped them to get through a very difficult time in their life. While I'm not usually a big fan of breaking things (I don't like to waste resources), this may be exactly what is needed, and you can make something beautiful with the broken pieces or donate them to an art center. Other common releases of anger include hitting a ball, chopping wood, needle felting, and running or other physical exercise. These exercises are beneficial when we cannot safely and appropriately direct our anger, such as when the situation is too big, you are about to hit rage, or you are releasing held anger.

Another trick I have learned is to send the fire of anger out to my aura. I let this fire cleanse and renew my aura until the fire has died down. When I do this, I feel more clear-headed and empowered, which is much better than internalizing the anger.

Anger causes the body to release and focus a large amount of energy, hence the urge for movement. This surge of energy can be an easy way to feel powerful. If we are not in alignment with our Integrity, we can become addicted to this feeling of power, which is a form of power over and domination. This power is an illusion. Many people in positions of power use their anger and rage as a way of maintaining their authority and worth. They know that the emperor is not wearing any clothes and so they hide behind the screen of ridiculous outbursts.

Eliciting anger is a great way of controlling people as well. Therefore, we need to be cautious when reacting to the media. Is this the full story? Is the story being slanted in a particular direction? Who gains from my anger? Is this how I want to spend my energy? When I find myself getting angry or overwhelmed by the media, I go outside and spend time with Nature. I say that I am going to get the "real news." Nature helps to put everything in perspective, offers me guidance, and reminds me of what is important. I do not want to be a cog benefitting a system that is not in alignment with Nature.

External and Internal Control

Dandelion reminds me to let go of control and to trust. Ki says, "When we let go of control, we enter into the flow. We move in alignment with Spirit."

Dandelion is talking about letting go of external control. When we use our force of will or techniques of manipulation to try to create a certain outcome, we exert external control. External control is particularly problematic if our efforts interfere with someone's free will. External control is restrictive and limiting and generally includes a component of fear. External control takes us out of alignment with our Soul and Nature.

External control is often a trauma response. When we are young there is much that we cannot control. If the adults in our life are explosive, we may learn how to create a situation that is least likely to elicit a negative reaction. Sometimes when we've experienced abusive childhoods or even adulthoods, we can lock ourselves in a box in the hopes of creating a safe environment. This box can look like our routines or even our daily practice. The box might not become apparent until we are in a new environment where we cannot set the parameters, for instance when we travel to a foreign country or when we collaborate on a project with someone for the first time.

Nature does not like rigidity. As Ani DiFranco says, "What doesn't bend, breaks."[3] We are meant to be flexible and open to Spirit and the energies around us. We think these boxes, our routines, our parameters are to keep us safe or to help us have a better life. But often they keep us from fully experiencing the world and life. An extreme version of this is agoraphobia, fear of leaving one's house. The truth is that these boxes are an illusion of control. Sooner or later, we will learn this lesson. The more we try to control, the more dramatic and painful the lesson.

Another aspect of external control is perfectionism and the belief that we have to do everything ourselves, that either no one else can do it as well as us or that no one else is willing to do it. This belief leads to exhaustion and, oftentimes, resentment.

I love my Nanny; she and my Pop-Pop, my paternal grandparents, are probably the people who taught me the most about unconditional Love. And my Nanny was a control-freak. I didn't notice this as a child, though the family joke was that Nanny cleaned with Q-tips (which was true). As an adult, I would (internally) chuckle at her control issues. For years, I visited on Tuesdays to take them food shopping and have lunch. Every week I would set the table and every week she would "fix" it. I knew how she liked it done and I did it that way, but it was not to her standards. I could give a long list of other examples. Years ago, I recognized how my grandparents made themselves sick from nervous tension, trying to fulfill their high expectations. This encouraged me to let go of my own high expectations. Nanny did not want to talk much about her childhood; but I do know that her father was abusive and extremely controlling. I am sure that her perfectionism was a residual effect from her childhood trauma of trying to make everything perfect to avoid her father's wrath.

I recognized my tendency toward control, perfectionism, and martyrdom when my children were toddlers. This became greatly apparent when I worked on projects with others and often ended up doing almost all of the work (of my own accord). Now I know that when I am starting to feel like a martyr ("I have to do everything around here!") or I'm trying to control a situation, I need to get curious. What is going on? What needs are not being met? Am I triggered? Am I stuck in an old story?

Letting go of external control can require much difficult (and sometimes scary) work. Again, control is a coping mechanism that most likely served us well in our lives, but now it is keeping us from experiencing the beauty of the world, our potential, and the gifts of others. Trying to control someone else (even with good intentions) prevents them from learning their lessons and experiencing the world and their gifts. When we shift away from this trauma response, we experience freedom and reduce our stress load. I think about the Dandelion seedheads floating in the wind—I can hear them giggling. In time, life becomes more enjoyable when we can go with the flow.

The COVID pandemic quickly demonstrated how little control we have over our lives. We can fight and try to hold onto control with everything we have. Or we can recognize the illusion and surrender. Contrary to what some think, surrender does not mean that we become powerless or give control to others. Instead, it is realizing that no one can control our lives—not even us. Surrendering allows us to move with the flow of life without resistance, saving us an enormous amount of time and energy and allowing everything to proceed more easily and smoothly. By becoming more conscious of our Soul Path and the energies around us, we are able to determine the best path forward.

While Dandelion encourages us to let go of external control, ki also teaches us to embrace internal control. When we learn how to work with energy, we discover the importance of internal control. Some refer to this as managing our emotions and reactions, understanding that while we cannot control our external circumstances, we can control our response. This is part of internal control, but not the complete story. Quantum physics demonstrates that we create the world and our lives. Therefore, if we want a certain experience, we work internally. We heal our wounds, we shed limiting beliefs, we remove blockages. And yes, we learn how to manage our emotions, respond from a Heart-centered calm, and trust that all is well (as often and as best as we can). In essence, we align ourselves with our Soul and with Nature. By doing this, we naturally move into the flow of the universe, which can translate to greater synchronicity and ease. By no means does this mean that we do not experience challenges or difficulties, but we are more able to navigate them.

Dandelion's seedheads take delight in letting go and dancing in the wind because they know that wherever they land, they will root and blossom. Ki invites us to let go of external control and embrace internal control so that we too can blossom wherever life takes us.

As I spend time with Dandelion, again and again I am reminded of the enormous amount of poison that we utilize every year to eradicate this amazing Plant. This desire to have weed-free lawns and gardens is connected to the belief that we need to control Nature. Dandelion asks, "When will humanity learn that they cannot control Nature and instead recognize the gifts that are being offered to them?"

We need to reevaluate our sense of beauty, for a large monocultural expanse of Grass is not found anywhere in Nature growing on ki's own. The mere idea is ludicrous. It requires a tremendous investment in time, energy, and poisonous chemicals while depriving us of the gifts Nature wants to share including food, medicine, and habitat for other species. One of the best things we have done at Heart Springs Sanctuary was to stop mowing large areas and to only mow paths through other areas. The bird population has greatly increased since then. Their songs fill our days with joy while our workload (and stress) has reduced. Getting rid of the perfectly manicured lawn opens the door to a life (and society) that is more aligned with Nature.

The more we try to control Nature (or really anything), the more out of control everything feels. What we are meant to learn in this is to let go and go with the flow. Dandelion helps us to stand in the place of not knowing, beckoning us to release, trust, and move in alignment with Spirit. When we are truly in alignment with Nature, we know that no matter what, we will be okay.

Seven Directions

When we are lost, Dandelion helps us to find our roots. Dandelion reminds us that wherever we are, we are a part of Earth, loved and nourished by ki. We navigate the world through the Seven Directions: East, South, West, North, Below, Above, and Center. They guide us through the events and stages of life and aid us in knowing where we stand and where we are heading. Sometimes we get stuck in a direction. Perhaps we had a serious breakup that we just can't seem to get over; we might need to move out of the West. If we find ourselves dreaming and visualizing but not able to complete any of our projects, we might be stuck in the East.

The Directions have different attributes in different traditions. We want to develop our own relationship with each direction so that we know them well. I am sharing the attributes that I work with simply as a starting point. These are based on attributes I've learned from the Reclaiming Tradition, Pam Montgomery, and I'm sure from other teachers I have worked with as well, but mostly these attributes reflect my own experiences with the Directions.

We start with the four cardinal directions. This is the plane where we walk and describes how we interact with the world. Refer to the chart on page 113 for the attributes of the cardinal directions.

Unfortunately, reading about these directions in a chart makes them seem flat and static, whereas the Seven Directions are living energies. When you get to know them, they each have their own distinct energetic impressions that are connected to your experiences and understanding of the world. Again, I encourage you to start your own investigation into the Seven Directions.

You might identify a direction that resonates with you or that is more difficult to connect with. It took me many years to be comfortable with the North. When I called in the Directions, I could identify many aspects for the East, South, and especially the West, but hardly any for the North. Of course, North was the Direction that I needed to connect with the most.

We connect to Source through the three vertical directions: Below, Above, and Center. Below is connected to Mother Earth. This is where many of the Plant Spirits live and where we go to connect with them. We visit the Underworld to access information, meet with our Spirit guides and helpers, and access our subconscious. The Below is connected to earthworms, mycelium, and other Beings who take the unwanted, the unneeded, and turn them into compost. Comfrey supports our connection with the Below.

ATTRIBUTES OF THE FOUR CARDINAL DIRECTIONS

Aspect	East	South	West	North
Element	Air	Fire	Water	Earth
Season	Spring	Summer	Fall	Winter
Time of Day	Dawn	Noon	Dusk	Midnight
Animal	Eagle, Hawk	Coyote, Salamander	Dolphin	Bear
Color	White, Lavender	Red, Orange	Blue	Black, Brown
Plant	Dandelion, Lavender	Fireweed, St. John's Wort	Cedar, Horsetail	Oak, Burdock
Lifecycle	Young Child	Teenager/ Young Adult	Adult	Crone
Plant cycle	Planting Seeds	Growing Green Beings	Harvesting	Dormancy
Other Aspects	Far Vision, New Beginnings, Birth, Second Chances, Visioning, Inspiration, Winds of Change, Breath of Life, Clear Communication, Poetry, Song	Passion, Playfulness, Childlike Innocence, Community, Abundance, Sexual Desire, Laughter, Pleasure, Joy, Courage, Action, Daring Relationships	Intuition, Close Vision, Ancestors, Divination, Emotions, Connecting with Elemental Beings, Moon, Ocean Tides, Ebb and Flow, Release, Going with the Flow, Self-reflection, Self-healing, Grief	Silence, Deep Wisdom, Deep Nourishment, Rest, Repose, Dreamtime, Hibernation, Meditation, Sharing Stories, the Wisdom of Elders, Contemplation, Bones, Stones, the Structure of All

The Above is connected to Father Sky. This is the place where we connect with the angelic Beings who guide and protect us and help us to remember our Divine origins. We also connect with the otherworldly or cosmic Beings in the Above. These Beings help to bring cosmic wisdom to Earth, helping us to evolve, to see with a broader perspective, and to remember that we are universal Beings. We visit the Above world to access other dimensions, gain a bigger picture, or meet with the Plant Spirits who live here. The Above is connected to the cosmos, including astrology. Angelica supports our connection with the Above.

Finally, we have the Center, the place where we are all connected, where we are One. This is the place of the Heart space connected to the Holy Heart and our own Heart, as well as Love, the greatest force there is. It is here in the Center that we connect with our True Self and our Wise One within. The Center is related to infinite possibilities, the hologram, mystery, and the element of ether or the space between spaces. Tulsi supports our connection to the Center.

Setting Sacred Space

Setting Sacred space enables us to create a container of safety and support. We want to do this before we engage with the Unseen world or do any deep work with Plants. There are many different methods for setting Sacred space, and you will come to know what feels best to you. I generally call in the Directions, which means that I take a moment to get settled into my body. I then turn to the East and say something like, "I call to the Guides and Guardians of the East and air, to you, Eagle and you, Hawk, to the winds of change and the breath of life, to poetry and song, to new beginnings and second chances, to you, Dandelion, to far visions and springtime energy, to the dawn awakening, I thank you and I welcome you to this space." I then turn to the South and say something similar, highlighting the attributes of the South. I repeat the process for the West, North, Below, Above, and Center.

When I no longer need the Sacred container, I thank the Beings of each direction for their assistance in reverse order (starting with the Center and ending with the East). I like to close by saying, "Stay if you will, go if you must. Hail and farewell."

On days that I see clients, I start the day with my prayers, then I smudge myself and my office, and set Sacred space. I leave this container up all day, smudging before and after each client. Generally, when I teach weekend workshops, we smudge and set the Sacred container at the very beginning and will close this circle at the end of the weekend. If I'm struggling with my writing or a project, I set Sacred space to help me more easily connect with the Plant Spirits and my other Guides. I often create Sacred space before making Love. If setting Sacred space is not something that you are familiar with, I encourage you to experiment by creating Sacred space before different activities and observing how this affects your experience.

Wild Food

Dandelion is an incredible nutritive and delicious wild food. We can eat all parts of Dandelion. The flowers are commonly made into fritters, pancakes, jelly, and wine. Usually, the young leaves are preferred for salads, though I marinate older leaves in a balsamic vinaigrette, which helps them to be more tender and less bitter. The leaves can also be added to soups, stir-fries, frittatas, or any place that you would use a dark leafy green. The roots are delicious roasted and turned into a tea.

Eating wild foods is one of the great pleasures of life. I love that I can go out in the yard and gather free food, gifts from Nature. Wild food tends to have a higher nutritive value than our commercialized, domesticated foods. Because wild food is inherently connected to the natural cycles, the Plants of a particular season offer us exactly what our bodies need at that time. For instance, the spring greens like Stinging Nettle, Dandelion, and Chickweed help to get our digestive and lymphatic systems moving as we transition from the more sedentary lifestyle and higher fat diet of winter. More than that, when we eat wild foods, we stimulate our ancestral memory.

Wild foods offer us a greater variety of flavor than typical modern foods (including domesticated vegetables), which highlight the salty and extremely sweet. Our beloved Dandelion, for example, tastes quite bitter. Bitter is missing from most of the modern diet (with the possible exception of beer) and yet bitter is a vital flavor. When we eat bitter foods, our salivary glands are activated and our body begins to excrete digestive juices, helping us to better assimilate the nutrients in our food. Bitter foods in general help to support our liver and gallbladder. They awaken us and help us to connect with life.

I encourage you to include wild edibles in your diet. You may not enjoy the taste of a wild food at first, but give them a chance; sometimes we need to retrain our taste buds. If you do want to forage for edibles, of course, it is important to be able to accurately identify edible Plants. Fortunately there are numerous guidebooks as well as foraging cookbooks to help you know how to identify and properly prepare the food.

We always ask permission before harvesting anyone (including garden Plants and animals). When you recognize that Plants are intelligent, you can engage their guidance in harvesting. Plants acknowledge their role in Nature and they understand the need for harvesting them. They generously give of themselves, if we ask. Asking permission, however, also means being prepared to hear no. You must learn how to discern and practice receiving it, even if you are not comfortable with it at first. It is disrespectful to harvest without asking permission. If a Plant says, "No," respect this. There could be numerous reasons for the no. Perhaps, for example, you misidentified the Plant and ki is not edible, or there are not enough of the Plant to allow for harvesting, or there is an animal who is dependent on this Plant.

If you receive a "Yes," then ask the Plant to show you who to harvest. I look to see if there is a leaf or a branch that seems sparkly or waving and this is who I harvest. I learned to never take more than 10 percent of a Plant population, and I prefer to err on the side of caution. If I'm foraging in a public place, I want to leave enough Plants that it is difficult to tell that someone foraged there. When foraging at our Sanctuary, I harvest more, especially with Plants like Mugwort or Nettles who quickly regenerate. Still, I leave plenty for the other animals and insects. When we harvest a Plant's roots, we are taking their life and often preventing them from regrowing. Therefore, prudence is necessary. Numerous Plants have become endangered from over harvesting. I rarely harvest roots, but if I do, the Plant must be prolific and a fast grower. If possible, we can spread the seeds of the Plant or only cut off a small part of the root. We want these Plants to continue to grow and support future generations and so we want to be good stewards, harvesting in alignment with what is best for all.

Of course, we always offer our gratitude for the generosity of the Plant we are harvesting. We will talk more about reciprocity in the following chapter.

Exercise: Plant Dieting

Plant dieting is a term used to describe several different experiences. For the purpose of this book, Plant dieting refers to ingesting various preparations of a Plant. We receive information and healing gifts when we ingest a Plant.

In the HEARTransformation Apprenticeship, we spend an afternoon dieting a Plant, experiencing one preparation after another. If we were dieting Dandelion, for example, we would eat a blossom, drink Dandelion leaf tea, eat marinated Dandelion leaves, take a couple drops of whole Plant tincture, drink Dandelion root tea, rub Dandelion oil on our body, taste a few drops of Dandelion glycerite, ingest a drop of Dandelion Essence, drink a little Dandelion wine, taste Dandelion honey, and ingest Dandelion oxymel, and I would transmit the energy of Dandelion Plant Spirit.

Please only engage in this practice with safe, edible Plants.

- Ask permission from your Plant ally to harvest a small amount.
- Take a small bite, chewing this slowly, allowing the Plant to release ki's components, noticing your body's reaction as you chew. How does your mouth feel? Do any emotions, sounds, memories, or images surface?
- Each Plant preparation offers a unique energetic perspective of a Plant. Consume as many different preparations as you can, preferably from different parts of your Plant ally. As you ingest each preparation, be sure to check in with your body. Notice how you respond. What is the energy of a particular preparation? Do you receive any information or sensations? You can experience one preparation after another, like we do in the HEARTransformation Apprenticeship, or you can also try one form of the Plant a day. Have fun finding new ways of ingesting your Plant.
- Above all, enjoy!

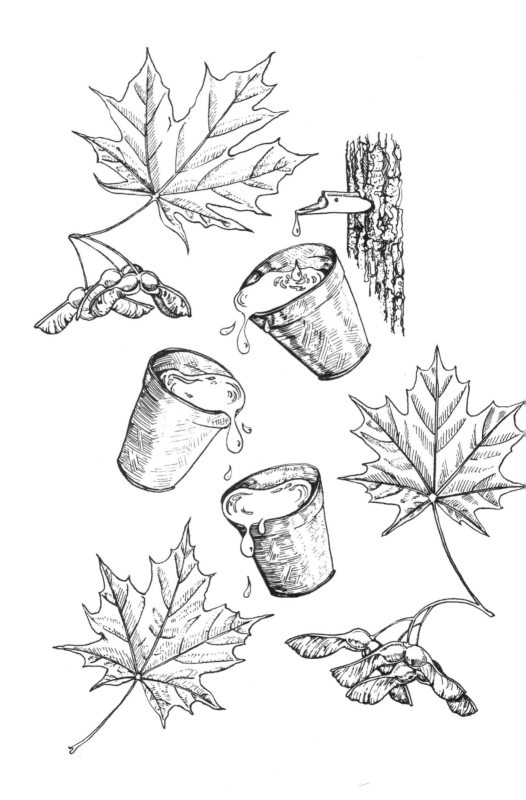

7
❧ Sweetness of Life ❦
Maple

When I moved to Heart Springs Sanctuary, the flowering Norway Maple radiated a green so vibrant that it had to be felt; it overwhelmed the eyes, the color of life and hope. How fitting since Maple provided medicine and nourishment to the Ancestors of this Land during the most dangerous time of year, providing hope that they had survived another winter and that the Green Beings would soon return. With grocery stores stocked year-round, we sometimes forget how precarious life once was in the late winter and early spring months.

Even now, the sweet momma's milk from Maple is one of life's great joys. Tapping Maple Trees brightens the often dark, gray days of winter. Such magic! You can put a tap into a Tree and collect sap that can be boiled down into delicious syrup. If you boil this even more, you get Maple sugar for candy or to spin for my family's favorite treat, Maple cotton candy. This extravagant deliciousness comes from a Tree and has been nourishing the people who lived here long before the colonists arrived. When we connect with Maple, we have the opportunity of remembering the potential of this Land, remembering how to live with Nature.

Generosity and Abundance

Maple pointed out ki's generosity to me during our first conscious conversation together: "We are your Elders, we have been here long before you, we came to this Earth long before you. We are generous. We feed many, we provide shelter for many. We live in true community. Learn from us. We gladly share our 'milk' with you; but ask first, show respect. We are generous, we will share, we want to be respected." Maple is an exceptionally generous Plant. Sharing ki's sap with us is only the beginning and yet that alone would make Maple a beloved Tree. If Maple grows near you, you know that in the spring they blanket the area with their helicopter seeds. I hear people express their disdain for this and I chuckle, for Maple is trying to help. A small Maple Forest quickly sprouted in the first area that we stopped mowing at Heart Springs Sanctuary. After three years, the Trees are a good size and the birds love them. They perch in the Forest and sing all day long. As Maple said, they provide food and shelter to many. Of course, Maple provides oxygen for us to breathe and consumes the carbon dioxide that we produce in excess. Ki's shade helps to cool us and the Earth, a much appreciated and necessary gift. The Maple that I sat with grew beside a creek and pointed out that ki helped to hold the soil. Maple adds much beauty to the world. When autumn arrives, Maple lights up the Land with ki's incredible colors. These leaves then fall and create more soil. And of course, Maple's wood, beloved of carpenters and craftspeople, provides warmth in winter. These are only a sample of Maple's many offerings.

Maple's generosity reminds us of the inherent abundance of Nature. If you've ever planted a seed or gardened you have tapped into this abundance. It amazes me that one Zucchini seed, for example, begets bushels of Zucchini, each containing hundreds of seeds. The abundance of Zucchini overwhelms, compelling you to share and encouraging you to enlarge your community to find those who are in need.

If our financial system was aligned with Nature's abundance, there would be no more poverty or hunger. But of course, that it is not aligned with Nature is the core issue with our financial system. Capitalism requires competition, which is created with the false belief of scarcity. Nature teaches us about abundance, cooperation, and the importance of diversity. Maple demonstrates that generosity is a vital component to the energetics of abundance.

When we align ourselves with Nature, we see the abundance that surrounds us, including food, medicine, beauty, guidance, and so much more. We see how Nature is there to help us whenever we need it. It is generosity that stimulates this abundance. When I get caught up in lack or not enough, that is my clue that I need to be more generous, that the energetics of abundance have become stagnant and I need to create a shift. The culture of capitalism teaches us to hoard. You will be successful and happy once you've accumulated a certain amount of money or things. The problem is that that amount is the elusive carrot on a string, always shifting so that you can never reach it. Hoarding does not bring us to abundance; it feeds lack, furthering the separation between us and others.

There is a difference between saving and hoarding. With the current social structure in the United States, it is important to save (if you can) for retirement, health crises, college, a house, and unforeseen circumstances. But there is a limit to how much money one needs (and if we changed the social structure, individuals wouldn't need as much as they do currently). If our financial system was aligned with Nature, we would not hoard. Imagine if our money spoiled like Zucchini. Rather than hoarding as much as we could, we would need to delight in the abundance as it was available, share the excess, and perhaps store some for the lean times. However, storing Zucchini requires effort, time, and space and there are limits to how long we can store ki, again encouraging us to share the abundance, enriching our lives through these relationships.

As we move into alignment with Nature, we reevaluate our needs and wants. Robin Wall Kimmerer writes in *Braiding Sweetgrass,* "In a consumer society, contentment is a radical proposition. Recognizing abundance rather than scarcity undermines an economy that thrives by creating unmet desires."[1] We are currently consuming resources at an unsustainable rate, leaving piles of trash and desecrated Land in our wake. Our amnesia mistook Nature's abundance and generosity, bringing out the worst in humanity as we raced to consume what we claimed was our inheritance. The word *consumption* can once again be connected to a deadly disease, though this time it is a psychological dis-ease, which may be more deadly than tuberculosis.

We are often told that we need to choose between our economy and the environment or Nature. However, if we look at the Greek roots of the word *economy*—*oikos* (house) and *nemein* (manage)—we see that the true meaning is "management of Home."[2] Therefore there is an inherent connection between the environment and our true economy. What contributes to a healthy environment contributes to a healthy economy. We've just been using the wrong metrics—money—to determine a healthy economy.

When we focus on money, we overlook the many facets of abundance in our lives. We also limit who can experience abundance. Money is merely a symbol, an extraction of Nature's currency of energy. Nature's currency has many forms including seeds, tools, handicrafts, food . . . the possibilities are endless. When we engage in a direct exchange, we honor the Sacred transaction that occurs. We want everyone involved to benefit and we understand that we each have an inherent value. This exchange is a way of feeding one another on multiple levels. When we substitute money, it is easy to forget the Sacredness of the exchange and to devalue one another, looking for a way to stretch our limited dollars. Suddenly everything has a price. A Tree, a river, a person can be exchanged for the right amount of money. This is short-sighted, because Nature's abundance is more than what can be extracted for monetary value. Often the most valuable aspects do not have a monetary value, like clean water, wild rivers, and intact Forests.

No one wants to be in a relationship with someone who endlessly takes and does not offer anything in return. When I invite people into my home, I tell them to make themselves comfortable, make themselves at home, help themselves to what they need. I don't expect that they will come in and take everything, leaving an empty shell, and nor would I do that to someone else. So why do we think that we can raid Earth? It's disrespectful not only to Earth, but to one another and future generations.

Maple invites us back to the Sacred cycle of giving and receiving. Ki tells me, "We provide homes to the bugs, to the birds. They provide meaning and purpose and beauty to us. They make our day brighter. . . . Take and receive, there must be a balance to this. We gladly give and are given to by others." In this we see that when we are aligned with Nature, we benefit both from the giving and the receiving.

Receiving is part of abundance. In order to be generous, someone needs to receive. I know many people who are happy to give and absolutely refuse to receive, acting as if receiving is a weakness. By doing so, they are not allowing someone else to express their gifts. When we graciously receive, we appreciate the unique offering of someone else, recognizing their beauty and their worth.

Ask for What You Want

As I write, I look out at the small Maple Forest that recently grew here. Only now do I see the gift in this and I am once again floored at the incredible generosity of the Plants. Our Sanctuary is located on a corner. While ki feels like a magical oasis, the Sanctuary is not as private as I had originally thought. I wanted to create areas where it felt completely safe to be vulnerable and to have ceremony without feeling like we were in a fishbowl. There are large White Pine Trees growing on the west side along the road. I pondered these and wondered how I could create a thicker screen, without finding a solution. During my check-ins with the Nature Spirits, I regularly made a request for more privacy. I now see that this Maple Forest is the answer to my requests. Ki creates a lovely screen that allows us to garden and hold ceremonies in peace, while also being serenaded by the birds. I thought that I was the one who was being generous by giving them this area to grow, but Maple was reminding me to ask for what I need and to let Nature provide.

Some of us have been taught that it is impolite to ask for what you want or that people who are close to you should be able to intuit what it is that you need. For many years, I believed that if I had to ask my then-husband for something, it became less special. I truly expected him to understand my needs without expressing them. After all, I was able to do this for others. I have since learned that this "skill" of intuiting others' needs is a trauma response that always had me on alert. After years of therapy, I finally realized that my husband truly didn't know what I wanted and it wasn't his responsibility to figure it out; I needed to express my desires. Now I excel at stating what I need and want.

When we work with Nature, we discover that ki (and really the universe) conspires to give us what we want. However, the possibilities are endless; therefore, it is helpful if we express our desires. Above all, Nature and Spirit want to give us what is in alignment with our Soul. If our desires are out of alignment, often they will not be provided. For instance, a luxury car most likely has no benefit for your Soul. You may make enough money to purchase one, but after a time you may discover that this car does not fulfill you, that now there is another longing for something else. Sometimes (or, in my case, often) Nature's timing is quite different from our own.

When expressing your desires, it is important to be as clear as possible without being limiting. For example, I asked to have privacy on the Land, especially for our ceremonies and gardening. I did not ask for a Maple Forest to grow. I didn't even consider this possibility. I expressed my need and allowed Nature to guide me in fulfilling this. Sometimes my input is required and other times, as in this case, Nature does all of the work.

Reciprocity

Maple asks, "What do you give, what do you bring to us?" When Nature provides our very life and shares so generously with us, our own gifts or offerings may seem minuscule. However, reciprocity is required; therefore, we give what we can. At the very least, we offer words of gratitude. Creator has given us a tongue so that we can speak (and sing) beauty into this world. When we are gifted something—a flower, words of wisdom, or Maple sap—we want to honor these gifts. Reciprocity helps us to engage in an exchange rather than taking. True to the cycle of giving and receiving, when we engage in reciprocity, we utilize the positive

Heart impulses of gratitude and appreciation. Reciprocity helps us move into our Heart space.

When we engage through the spirit of reciprocity, we open ourselves to a more beautiful world. Suddenly we see the abundance of gifts surrounding us; we are more fully able to appreciate the immense wonders of Earth. Reciprocity is not a balancing of ledgers or a rote thank you card. It is recognizing that our very life is dependent on the other Beings with whom we share this Earth. Reciprocity is a state of being.

As I mentioned in the last chapter, whenever we harvest, we always give an offering. That offering should be something that is meaningful to you and/or the Being you are giving it to. Many people think of the gifts of Cornmeal and Tobacco. These are beautiful offerings and the traditions of many Indigenous Nations; however, do they have meaning to you? Corn and Tobacco are Sacred Plants who are grown with prayers and song, then harvested with prayers and song. Corn is ground into Cornmeal. Have you ever ground Corn, by hand? It requires time and energy and of course, more prayers and songs. Offering Cornmeal that you have grown, harvested, and ground is more meaningful than going to the store and buying Cornmeal off a shelf.

During the Plant Spirit Healing Apprenticeship, Pam Montgomery taught us to gift beads, a tradition that comes from Martín Prechtel. A human exerts effort to create a bead, drilling the hole. In the HEARTransformation Apprenticeship, my students make their beads out of clay. I prefer working with clay because it will biodegrade into soil. As we make them, we add our prayers of gratitude. Again, making your own bead has more meaning than buying one in the store.

There are numerous ways to engage in reciprocity. Sometimes we show our gratitude by sharing the Plant's gifts or teachings with others. We sing or dance for a Plant. We write a poem. We make a beautiful piece of artwork. We gift food or drink. We give a Plant our breath, water, or our blood. We might plant other Plants nearby or clear debris. Sometimes we need to protect or speak up for a Plant (or other Being). When in doubt, ask the Plant what ki would like.

The point is that we give back. Reciprocity feeds Spirit, especially our own. Perhaps the best way to show reciprocity is to live a life of beauty that is aligned with Nature and our Souls, allowing every action to be an act of reciprocity, feeding the world with our own unique gifts.

There is a sense among some that humans are a parasite on the Earth and the best thing that we can do is to leave Nature alone or, even more extreme, to kill ourselves. All Beings, including humans, have a vital role to play in Nature. We can engage in reciprocity while we are discovering our role. Perhaps reciprocity will even help us remember.

Sweetness of Life

There is a common belief that life is difficult and we must work hard for anything worth having. However, Maple reminds us that this is human conditioning. We can focus on the sweetness of life just as easily as we focus on life's difficulties. This is not to say that we want to fly around with our feet barely touching the Earth, trying to avoid or ignore anything challenging. However, our frame of reference (including our beliefs) greatly influences what we experience and what we can see.

I can act as if cooking dinner is an act of suffering or I can delight in the incredible foods that I am working with, thinking about their origins as Plants and animals, thinking about the farmers and all the other Beings who brought them to my kitchen. I can use the act of cooking as a way of honoring these Beings while creating nourishment for myself and my family. I can put music on and dance and sing and fill this food with Love and joy, knowing that my family will ingest these qualities. I typically enjoy cooking, so it is easy for me to give this example. I also have days when cooking feels like a chore, when I don't feel well or I'm focused on a project. Those days, I generally do not cook; we eat leftovers, my partner cooks, we get takeout, or we make sandwiches. I realize that I am privileged to have options. However, the point is that with every act we do, we have a choice—we can treat it as a form of suffering or a form of joy.

The Plants have taught me not to engage in gardening when I feel that it is a chore. If I did, I would infuse the garden with the energy of suffering. Now when the garden begins to feel like a burden, I know that I have been working too hard and need to remember the sweetness of life.

Everyone has challenging moments (sometimes lasting for years). If we are able to look up in the midst of them, we can find beauty. This is as simple as focusing on your breath and remembering that this air is given to you by the Plants. When we live a life aligned with Nature, we discover that we are never alone in our suffering, that we are surrounded by Love and guidance. Giving ourselves even a few minutes in Nature can help to ease the burden and bring a smile to our faces.

Sometimes trauma, especially childhood trauma, can make life feel as if every day is another torturous act. Fortunately, we can heal from trauma. While we are in the process of recovery, Maple helps us to shift our point of view to see the joy that surrounds us. If we continue to process our trauma and connect with Nature, we will eventually be realigned with the sweetness of life.

I have witnessed people afraid to delight in life. They are concerned that if they are too happy, something bad will happen. (This is a trauma response and based on a limiting belief.) Or they feel guilty because other people are dealing with atrocities. We do not help anyone by lessening our joy and enjoyment of life. When we express joy or happiness, we radiate this energy, adding these experiences to the collective energy. More than that, our enjoyment honors the many Beings who support us, becoming another form of reciprocity. I consider joy and pleasure as an investment; I want to thoroughly saturate myself with these experiences to give me a boost for the challenges of life. If I do not allow myself to experience joy, I reduce my resiliency.

As a wise one once told me, "You need to remember the frame." If everything is a struggle and a chore, then something needs your attention. Perhaps we just need to readjust the frame or clean the glass. And sometimes we need to change systems of oppression. When life is good and we are able to bask in its sweetness, we can remember Maple's other message about supporting one another. Look around—can you reduce someone's suffering or give them a boost so that they too can enjoy the sweetness? Remember, we thrive together.

Nourishing Ourselves

Some of us have been taught to think of others first, taking care of their needs at the expense of our own. Society rewards (and often expects) selfless acts, especially when it comes to parenting. Of course, a young child requires a lot of energy and attention and it is not appropriate to expect them to take care of their own needs. However, our culture is designed so that the weight of this falls on the shoulders of the parents, often primarily on just one parent. Ideally, the raising of a child should be a communal affair where family members, friends, and even professionals support the child and their parents so that their needs are met with Love. Parenting a young child is only one example of where we might be expected to ignore our own needs. This can happen in a work environment, a relationship, or when caring for a family member. Of course, there are those who seem to be the perennial doormat, who often do not even know what their needs are. Too often, those of us who were taught to take care of others' needs surround ourselves with people who seemingly have an insatiable need and are oblivious to our limitations and requirements.

When we sacrifice our needs for someone or something else, we cause an energy drain and we move out of Integrity. If we do this too often, we find ourselves depleted, which can ultimately lead to serious dis-ease and sometimes even death. Along the way, there are warning signs trying to get our attention. Stress, irritability, exhaustion, weepiness, and physical discomfort are some of the possible signs. Ideally, we recognize these signs and take the time to fill ourselves again. Sadly, there is a tendency to only recognize what is happening when we have reached a crisis level.

For many years, I was a stay-at-home mom, homeschooling my children, designing and building our homes, managing a large homestead, frequently helping my grandparents, running a small herbal and Flower Essence practice, assisting numerous friends and family members, and supporting my then-husband and his business in countless ways. On top of this, I was a vegetarian and, in hindsight, was not receiving the physical nourishment that I needed, especially during the six years that I was pregnant and nursing. I rarely had time for myself, and when I did, I was usually doing something to benefit my family or my growing healing practice. When my husband came home from work, I would fairly regularly say that I just needed fifteen to twenty minutes, and would go in my room and cry. I was trying to rest and center myself, but we lived in a tiny house and I could hear that my family needed me, so I would soon return without filling myself.

Eventually this led to Lyme disease, which only intensified my experience. Now I was continually exhausted and frequently in pain, while still trying to accomplish everything that I did before even though the simplest task, like hanging up laundry, completely exhausted me. I honestly am not sure how I made it through.

About five years after contracting Lyme disease, I was sitting in my Flower Essence training with David Dalton and Kate Gilday when David said something that changed my life. He said that a major contributing factor to Lyme disease is someone who puts more energy out than they bring in. All of the lights and whistles went off—this was me. True to my nature of wanting to support others, I suddenly had the realization that if I wanted to be able to help my kids, friends, and family members, I needed to take care of my own needs first. This was absolutely revolutionary to me. I was always the last on my list and usually was too exhausted to get to me.

Since that class, I have made my needs and wants a priority. I know that I am a better person, mother, partner, and healer when I am fulfilled. Sure, my old habits kick in sometimes and I start dropping the activities that support me, like spending time in Nature or with friends, dancing, or even my morning rituals. But often I do this consciously for a short time period and then schedule an extended time afterward for me to do what I want. Or, if I wasn't conscious of it, I at least start to recognize the signs early and then quickly stop and go be with the Plants. The signs for me are that I get stressed, I start feeling like the world is doomed, or I feel irritable, maybe even get snappy with my loved ones.

Maple reminds us that nourishing ourselves is vital to our thriving. Of course, what nourishes you may be different for others. If you put others' needs before your own, you may not even know what your needs are. Take time to discover them and to try new experiences. Our needs may change over time. When my kids were younger, I delighted in going to a restaurant by myself. I would bring a book and eat and read in silence for an hour or so, a very rare occurrence for me. Now that my children are grown, I much prefer to have dinner with them.

Recently there has been much focus on self-care. Self-care can be a part of nourishing ourselves, but they are not synonymous. Sometimes people utilize a self-care regimen to enable them to continue with a job or a relationship that is draining and ultimately not in alignment with their life. Despite their acts of self-care, they are not in Integrity. The ideal situation is that the majority of our life is set up to nourish us, down to the smallest details, while knowing that there will be times that will require more from us, such as when a loved one dies.

While you are discovering what nourishes you, pay attention to how your daily activities affect you. Get into your Heart space and feel how your body is responding. Does it uplift you (ping) or deplete (thud)? You may have some activities that are depleting, perhaps commuting to work or doing the dishes. Again, this is about balance. Can you do something to lessen the depletion? Perhaps you work from home a couple days a week or you commute with a co-worker you enjoy, or you listen to audiobooks by your favorite authors. Sometimes we need to drop depleting activities and sometimes we can shift them so that they are less depleting or even fulfilling. The key is to know how they affect us.

Activities do not always fit into distinct categories of nourishing or depleting. For instance, teaching a weekend class absolutely fills my Heart and Soul, and I am often physically exhausted at the end. I have noticed some changes that I can make to lessen the depletion including having a teaching assistant or work-study students, hiring someone to cook the meals, lessening the preparations needed, and having a quiet space to go to for breaks and at the end of the day. I have implemented some of these and am working on shifting others. In the meantime, I schedule a day or two after teaching for rest and spending time in Nature.

A great way to start or add to a commitment to nourish yourself is to create a daily practice. This can consist of whatever fills you and can be as short as five minutes or as long as a couple of hours depending on your needs and life situation. For years my daily practice consisted of smudging, calling in the Directions, giving an offering to the Faeries, doing Sun Salutations or dancing, and walking the Labyrinth or the Land. My practice changed when my Beloved joined my life. Now we share our dreams, read to one another, and make tea before I engage with some of my other practices. On days when I am seeing clients or feel that I need support, I smudge and call in the Directions. This morning practice sets the tone for the rest of the day. How would you like to start your days?

Exercise: Engaging in Reciprocity with Your Plant Ally

Your Plant ally has offered you many gifts, even before you started to communicate with them. Now it is your turn to give to them.

- Ask your Plant ally what ki would like. If you are unsure, tune into your Heart and see if something comes forward.
- When you have the gift, present this to your Plant friend.
- Speak your prayer of gratitude aloud to your Plant ally as you present your gift. Remember all the many ways in which ki has supported you (and others). Knowing that your act of reciprocity feeds the Plant Spirit, be sure to offer ki your most nourishing, sweetest words of Love. We speak these words of beauty aloud so that they may affect the vibration of the wind and reverberate throughout the Earth.
- Feel free to repeat this exercise. You can engage in reciprocity with your Plant ally again and again.

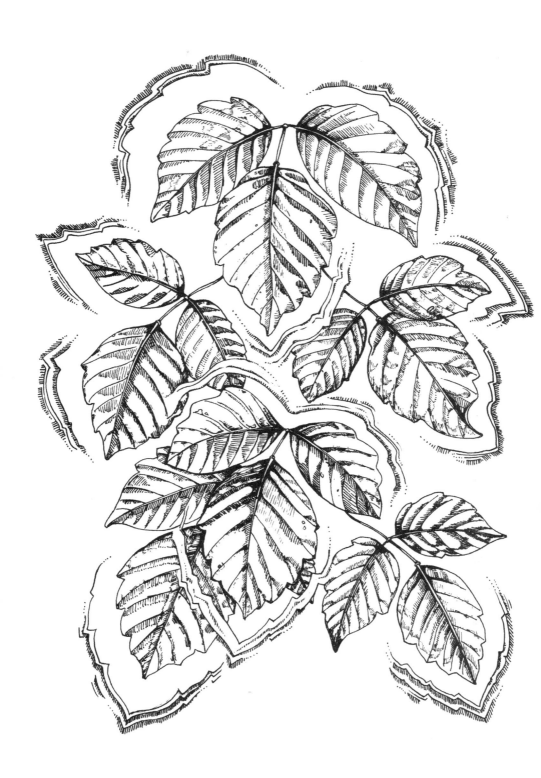

8
❧ From Foe to Friend ❧
Poison Ivy

*P*oison Ivy. Simply hearing the name causes some to itch. This is
possibly one of the most known and despised Plants, at least in
the United States. Even young children are taught, "Leaves of three,
let them be." And yet, Poison Ivy is one of my Beloveds. (To be fair,
I have not experienced the horrendous rash that most get when they
come into contact with ki.) I tend to refer to Poison Ivy as Sister
Protectress, which highlights one of ki's great skills. Many of my students have also fallen in Love with Sister Protectress and others at
least have an improved if still cautious relationship—one student even
got a tattoo of Sister Protectress. Regardless of your prior beliefs about
Poison Ivy, if you can enter into innocent perception and be willing
to spend time with ki, Sister Protectress has wisdom to share, and you
too may fall in Love.

Boundaries

The famous saying about Poison Ivy demonstrates one of ki's incredible
teachings. When you see Sister Protectress, leave ki be. Do not enter
or at least proceed at your own risk. Sister Protectress teaches us about
boundaries. Sadly, having good boundaries is not a skill that we teach

children. In fact, we tend to ignore the boundaries of children, which can set them up for a lifetime of poor boundaries, either ignoring their own or not respecting those of others. I frequently guide my clients in learning how to set good boundaries—or even recognizing that they are allowed to have them. Often when I first mention boundaries to them, they look kind of dazed, unsure of what that even means. We start by regularly checking in with themselves, "Is this mine? Or does this belong to someone else?" We also work on learning how to distinguish their energy from someone else's. Essentially, a boundary is a meeting point, a place where something (a person's aura, a meadow, a building) ends and something else begins. More than that, a boundary is a limit that can look like a set of rules or agreements about what you are willing to accept or do.

Boundaries might look like stating: I will only work late one night a week, I will come in early and leave at 4 p.m., I do not answer emails on weekends, I turn my phone off at 9 p.m. They may also include statements like I do not drink alcohol when I drive, or I have complete body autonomy and only engage in sexual activities when and how I want, even in a partnered relationship. There are many more examples. Please refrain from name-calling when talking to me. I do not like to be touched there. This is the price. I am taking a mental health day. I do not eat sugar. I am allergic to nuts. I need time to process and will respond next week. No shoes, no service.

Boundaries help to keep us safe, protect our energy, and teach others how we want to be treated. Nourishing ourselves and making our needs a priority are important boundaries. Saying "No" creates a boundary. Learning about boundaries is especially important for empaths. They often feel things that are not theirs and, therefore, are not their responsibility. Being able to distinguish what is mine and what is not mine saves quite a lot of energy and emotional turmoil.

Our auras provide a natural boundary for us. When they are healthy, they help to filter and reject anything that is not in service of us: illnesses, negative energies, radiation, ill intentions, and so much more. Unfortunately, our auras are often overwhelmed by the pollution (including energetic and emotional pollution) that surrounds us. When we engage in energy hygiene, we clear and strengthen our auras.

Our auras are incredible. They adjust depending on our surroundings and our physical, mental, emotional, and spiritual states. In general, they are a bubble that is about one arm's length away from our body in all directions (including below our feet). When we are in a stressful situation, such as a near accident, our auras contract. This is a way of protecting our energy. We can expand our auras in meditation and similar activities, sometimes making them quite large. To get a sense of your aura, extend your arms and feel all around you. It may help to be in your Heart space and to close your eyes. What do you feel? Is there an area that is warmer or cooler? Do any colors come to mind? Can you feel some resistance on your hand? If so, you are meeting the boundary of your aura. If you are struggling with this, rub your hands together first, feeling the warmth and energy you are creating, and then reach out toward the edges of your aura. Or engage your imagination; if you were to sense your aura, what color would it be?

Having good boundaries helps us to have a strong aura. The more we ignore our boundaries, the more difficult it is to maintain a healthy aura, making us more susceptible to illnesses, negative energies, and ill intentions. Again, balance is important. Sometimes our boundaries can become a jail, keeping us from truly enjoying life. The energetic feeling is rigidity. If you are recovering from trauma, you may need to have stronger boundaries until you can feel safe. As you heal, you may discover that some boundaries are no longer needed. You may also find that you need to have firmer boundaries with some people or in certain situations.

The term *boundaries* is sometimes misused to excuse judgment and divisiveness. Usually this is because people do not actually have good boundaries, so they set up a fortress. Unfortunately, this fortress feeds the separation myth and limits their experiences. For example, I do not engage in dialogue with people who have different political beliefs, or I don't date people from a different religion, or, a common one on social media, If you believe _____, unfollow me are not boundaries. These are judgments that deny the humanity of other people and eliminate the possibility of connection. Poison Ivy does not say only people who are 6'4" can walk past me or only registered Green Party members can enter these Woods. Poison Ivy asks for a certain behavior: can you be observant and respectful? Or ki simply says, "This area needs to heal, please keep out." We need to be mindful of whether our boundary serves us (and the other party) or if it's a judgment. If we find that we are being judgmental or divisive, we can get curious. What is behind this? Usually, it is fear or trauma. This is an invitation to heal and discover new possibilities for engaging with people. Often this is also a sign that your aura needs some help—maybe you need to take some time out to focus on filling up and moving into your Heart space.

Setting a boundary is one thing; having your boundaries respected is another. If you have been a people pleaser, a martyr, an overachiever, an empath, or a doormat, you may discover that people keep testing your boundaries or that they do not respond well to you expressing your boundaries. It is possible that you are not expressing your boundaries as clearly as you may think you are. It is up to you to enforce your boundaries and if someone is not able to respect them, then you need to decide if you want to continue to be in relationship with them or if you are going to change your boundaries. Some types of people abhor boundaries, including narcissists, sociopaths, and people who are deep in their addictive behaviors. They will stomp all over your boundaries or manipulate you so that you feel bad when you attempt to enforce them. They will also slowly chip away until you find yourself without a boundary. For instance, if you tell a narcissistic ex-partner that they are not welcome at your home, they might drop a birthday gift off at the edge of your property, ask if they can give something to your kids, or want to deliver your support check themselves because it would arrive late if they mailed it. In my experience, it is best to have a very firm, clear boundary with them. Do not give an inch (especially if you do not feel safe around them)—they do not actually recognize compromise. You are not responsible for them, their emotions, or their previous actions that required you to set the firm boundary.

If you need help, you can always call on Poison Ivy. Ki knows how to set clear boundaries with consequences when these are not respected. You can ask Poison Ivy to surround your aura with protection or to create a shield around your house, or you can ask Poison Ivy directly for help setting strong, clear boundaries.

It can feel uncomfortable when we begin to set boundaries, especially if we are used to being a doormat. Setting normal, appropriate boundaries can feel as if we are being rigid and unreasonable, or even offensive to someone. We may feel as if we are being too demanding. It may be helpful to imagine how we would feel if the roles were reversed or to share our experience with someone who has healthy boundaries. If we pause and reflect, we may find that we feel empowered because we are no longer leaking energy. In time, setting boundaries becomes easier and even instinctive.

When we look to Nature, we see that boundaries are often the most diverse areas because there is a mixing of ecosystems. We can remember that by setting boundaries, we invite creativity and help all involved to flourish. In time, you will notice how much happier you are because of your boundaries, and it will become easier to express them.

Power of Saying No

No is a powerful word. Many of us are uncomfortable with these two letters. Either we do not want to be told "No," so we do not even ask or try. Or we are afraid to say "No" to others and let them walk all over us or do things that we do not want to do. Or both. This was me. I was terrified of having someone say no to me. I would only ask for something that I knew I was guaranteed to get. I truly thought that I would die if I was rejected. I did not like to disappoint anyone—I was a people pleaser, so I rarely said no. I would go way beyond my limits and do things that I didn't want to do because I felt obligated, which then led to resentment.

Years ago, a friend hosted a girls' night. My friend is incredibly talented and operates several businesses. While we were having fun cooking dinner together, one of the women asked if she could buy something from my friend. My friend said, "No." That was it. Later she said, "You can get it tomorrow if you like." I remember being stunned, but not because my friend was mean—there wasn't any emotion or charge in her response. I didn't know you could say no clearly without having to explain or feel bad. The woman who made the request seemingly wasn't asking for a lot; however, it would have required my friend to leave everyone else to focus on her work. My friend's response not only allowed her to stay focused on our gathering, it was also an invitation to the other woman to focus on and appreciate the present moment and to respect my friend's time. Clearly this left an impact, as I still think of it over ten years later. Those two letters were a gift in many ways.

Saying no is a lot easier for me now. I recognize that when I do this, I am saying yes to me and my boundaries. I'm also being honest with my relationships and preventing resentment. When the Plants tell me no, I'm grateful. I want to be respectful and in harmony with them. The same is true with my friends, clients, and family. I also ask for what I need and want, knowing that if I get a negative response, I will survive. There are worse things in life than being told no. I may be disappointed. But if it is really something that is in alignment with my Soul, I will find a way. "No" has saved me from many situations where I would have been unhappy, leading me to things that were better than I could ever have imagined. Sister Protectress willingly helps us learn how to both receive and say no.

Nature Reclamation

People have strong feelings regarding Sister Protectress. They seemingly do not appreciate ki's boundaries or perhaps they do not understand that ki is setting a boundary. If we pay attention and listen, we notice that Sister Protectress often grows in areas that have been abused and need reclamation. This is one way of keeping humans out so that Nature can heal. Sometimes Sister Protectress grows around Sacred areas, again to keep destructive humans out. Humans tend to think that we should be able to go wherever we want, but sometimes we aren't wanted there. When I see Poison Ivy growing, I sit with the Land to see what is needed. I ask Sister what ki is doing. Even if it feels like I can proceed or if I see a way in, I always ask permission before entering.

When I lived on the farm, I attempted to create a Sacred grove for ceremonies. Within weeks after planting the Trees, Sister Protectress started growing in the area, even though ki wasn't growing nearby. I thanked Sister and said that we did not need ki's service, that I would protect this area. After all, this Sacred site was created for humans to interact with Nature. Sister left the area.

At Heart Springs Sanctuary, we have several areas of Poison Ivy. I have discovered that they sometimes need to be cleared. Since I have yet to have a reaction, this is my job. It may sound like it is a misery to clear Sister, but I'm grateful when I get to spend time with ki. I ask before I clear any of the vine and I ask ki to direct me in the process. From this I have learned that not only is Poison Ivy teaching us how to respect boundaries, ki is helping us to set them. We have pathways throughout the Sanctuary and Sister started growing into several of them. I told ki that I needed humans to be able to walk through these without fear or getting hurt and so I needed to clear ki. Sister was happy that I set the boundary and then showed me how to enforce it. This is co-creative partnership in action. Listening to Nature and also explaining what we need so that we can work together.

Start Small and Be Humble

The first time that I worked with Sister Protectress at Heart Springs, I was clearing ki from a Sweet Gum Tree, which felt a little daunting. There were decently sized vines growing up the trunk and extending into the grass around the Tree. I thought that I should start with the large vines. Sister told me to start small, highlighting a very small Plant in the grass. I gently pulled this and as I did, more and more of the vine started to come out so that I was easily clearing the larger vines. I kept starting with a small part and soon the area and the trunk were clear. Amazing! Sister reminded me to start with one small step at a time.

Another time we were creating a new path to the ponds. I removed Poison Ivy and saw that there was a small Plant near where people would cross the creek and enter the path. I asked to clear this and ki said, "No, people need to learn to pay attention to their surroundings and to be humble." Ki was right, and I left the Plant there.

In the spirit of humility, I want to be clear that even though I have yet to have a reaction, I remain respectful of Sister. I know what ki is capable of. I cover my arms and legs (if exposed) with crushed Jewelweed (known to help prevent Poison Ivy rash). I then put reused plastic bags over my hands. I have used plastic gloves as well, but I prefer the bags. I am extremely careful when I pull the vines, though I still get whacked by them. I speak words of Love and gratitude and ask for guidance. When I am finished, I rub more crushed Jewelweed on any exposed areas, and for the next two days I take cold showers, being on the look-out for any potential rash.

If you are not so fortunate, Jewelweed may be your best friend. If you see Jewelweed growing, pause and look around the area, for there is a high chance that you will see Poison Ivy or Stinging Nettles as ki usually grows near them. (Jewelweed also helps with the sting and rash from Nettles.) French green clay or another powdered clay combined with apple cider vinegar to make a paste is incredibly helpful for a Poison Ivy rash. Cover the rash with the paste and let it dry completely then rinse with cold water, being sure to not rub it. Repeat every few hours until the rash clears. And perhaps, ask Sister Protectress what lesson ki would like to share with you.

From Foe to Friend

I can't say that I ever hated Poison Ivy. I think I mostly had a non-relationship with ki and was rather fearful. As I worked with the Land and came to understand Poison Ivy's role, I started to respect ki and with my new understanding our separation lessened. As I learned how to avoid the rash and the remedies that lessened the severity, my fear dwindled. In time I was able to recognize the beauty of Sister

Protectress. This allowed me to learn from ki and ultimately to truly love Poison Ivy. Now when I see ki growing, my Heart brightens and I thank ki for the incredible gifts that Sister Protectress brings to this Earth.

Sister didn't change who ki was; ki simply continued to protect and heal the Earth. I changed. My new perspective and Love helped me to strengthen my connection to Sister Protectress, the Land, and Earth. This is one more step in remembering my role as part of Nature. The more we know about where we live, the more we become a part of our special place, healing the separation.

This shift can be true for our human relationships as well. Too often we distance ourselves because of fear or misunderstanding. When we take the time to get to know someone or to hear their story, we often see their beauty. Once this occurs, they can no longer be a "foe" or feared. We may not agree with them or want to spend every day with them (I love to work with Sister, but I do not want to clear ki every day), but we can be grateful that they are a part of this Earth and perhaps even Love them.

Exercise: Drawing Your Plant Ally

The mention of something artistic may make you want to quickly turn the page, or maybe it excites you! For many of us, our school experience injured our innate artistic self. Please, have no worries—this activity is between you and your Plant. There are no grades and, of course, no judgment. I assure you that you are capable of doing this. You may find that you actually enjoy drawing with your Plant ally.

Drawing a Plant is an opportunity for close observation. We often see without really seeing. When we look closely at a Plant we discover patterns, different shapes, or bizarre forms that we previously missed, even if this is a Plant we've known for years.

For this project you may want paper, pencil, crayons, pastels, colored pencils, charcoal, a magnifying glass or loupe, and any other art supplies you enjoy working with. If you are uncomfortable with drawing, then charcoal, crayons, or pastels are great tools to start with.

🌿 To begin, sit with your Plant and move into your Heart center. When you are there, look at the forms and shape of your Plant. Use the magnifying glass or loupe to look closely at the flowers. As you are looking, be sure to share your amazement and appreciation with your Plant.

🌿 We begin with a gesture drawing. What do you feel or sense as you sit with this Plant? Are there dominant colors? Is there an energetic movement? Try to capture this. I prefer to use pastels or crayons for this drawing. This is a somewhat abstract, feeling drawing, not a detailed botanical illustration. If you showed this to someone, they probably wouldn't be able to tell you who you are working with, but would get a sense of the energy or feeling of this Plant.

🌿 You may want to make several gesture drawings, or maybe make them during different life cycles of the Plant or at different times of day.

🌿 The next step is a contour drawing. I like to use charcoal for this, but a pencil, marker, or crayon also works. For this kind of drawing, once you begin, keep your pencil on the paper the entire time, only lifting it when the drawing is complete. Keep your eyes on your Plant, not looking at the paper.

🌿 Looking at your Plant, choose where you would like to begin your contour drawing. Place your pencil onto the paper and draw the outline of the Plant, remembering to keep your eyes on the Plant and your pencil on the paper.

🌿 When you are finished, look at your paper. Can you see your Plant ally? This process often makes me laugh, and yet most of the time my drawing actually resembles the Plant. I say "actually" because I always wanted to create beautiful botanical drawings; I could see the images, but they got lost when I tried to translate them to paper. My friend Eli Weaver introduced me to contour drawing during one of her botanical drawing classes. I was amazed that I created something that looked like a Plant. One of my big lessons from this experience was that in order to create a recognizable drawing, I needed to relax and have fun.

🌿 If you would like, you can continue by creating a detailed botanical sketch, painting, or other artwork. Draw with your Plant as much as you like. If the Plant gives you permission, you can also trace a leaf or do a rubbing.

- Pay attention and note any revelations or sensations that occur as you are intently observing and drawing your Plant ally.
- Have fun and be sure to thank your Plant.

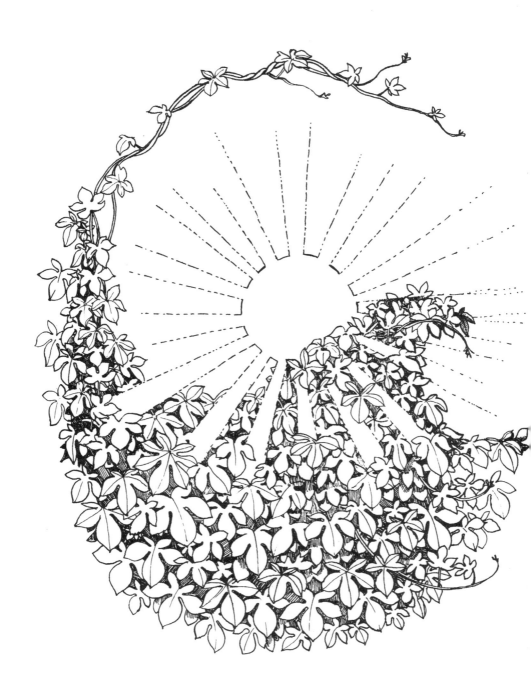

9
❧ Taking Action ❧
Japanese Hops

*J*apanese Hops are a fairly new Plant friend for me. They appeared the second year that I lived at Heart Springs Sanctuary. The following year this vine grew all over the Sanctuary. I knew that ki wanted to talk but I was too busy and did not have time. When I walked the Land to offer my prayers in the morning, ki would trip me, leaving brush burns on my legs. It really felt like ki jumped out of nowhere and grabbed my ankles. Japanese Hops is an "invasive" Plant that can easily pull down Trees. Japanese Hops moved in, covering large Elderberry Bushes, climbing White Pine and bending the branches, and completely covering the area that was formerly a dump.

When I wouldn't sit with Japanese Hops, ki got the attention of my students, telling them that ki wanted to talk to me. Still, I was overwhelmed and simply did not have the time. Japanese Hops continued to grow and grow until I finally had to create time. (Ki can grow over thirty feet in a single year, in many directions.)

No Such Thing as Invasive

As I sat with Japanese Hops, I felt an energy like a general marching their army across the Land. For the first time, I had a negative reaction to an invasive Plant. I know that people have strong opinions regarding so-called invasive Plants. Even people who are passionate defenders of Earth, who do not want any animal or insect to die, suddenly delight in the destruction of species they view as invasive. I, however, defend and befriend these species. Japanese Hops was showing me the intense fear that is associated with invasive Plants and testing my ability to look beyond the fear.

The Earth continues to evolve. With human destruction of the environment (and, I think, an increase in consciousness), the Earth is evolving more rapidly than ever before. We like to think that evolution occurred a long time ago and that everything is static now, but that's not accurate. It is readily apparent that the Earth is shifting; just look at the extreme weather or Forest fires. Plants continue to evolve with humanity, moving with us as we migrate. Many of our beloved Plants are not "native." The question I ask is what determines a native Plant? After frequently asking this question, I've discovered a couple responses. One is that native Plants have grown in an ecosystem for hundreds or thousands of years and were not introduced by humans. Another common response is that in the United States, native Plants are Plants who grew here before the colonists arrived.

I have serious issues with these definitions. They seem to discredit the enormous amount of gardening and Plant introduction that occurred in the United States before the colonists arrived and seem to forget that humans are a natural part of the ecosystem. Plants are designed to spread and be moved around. Some, like Burdock, have hooks on their seedheads to get caught on fur and clothing and then dispersed elsewhere. Others, such as Raspberry, surround their seeds in delicious flesh to entice animals (including humans) to eat them and excrete the seeds, spreading them far from the parent Plant. It could even be argued that the purpose of Plants' bright colors and gorgeous flowers is to attract people as well as pollinators, encouraging us to grow them. In Plant circles there is often a discussion about who is gardening whom? Are we gardening Plants or are Plants gardening us? In my case, the Plants definitely garden me.

Now before you start writing me nasty letters about how I'm going to destroy the Earth by allowing invasive species to grow, please hear me out. The ideal is to have Plants growing who contribute to the health of the ecosystem. Many of the native Plants have developed a longtime relationship with pollinators, birds, and other species in an area; but they are not always the best Plants for a specific area. Every year I spend time with the Beings who support the Sanctuary (I often refer to them as Faeries or Nature Spirits). I ask about the projects for the year and what Plants we should add. If there are Plants that I would like, I ask if we can plant them. Together we create a long list of Plants and then I find them. This list is a mixture of Plants: Trees, Bushes, annuals, perennials, so-called natives, naturalized, exotics, edibles, medicinals, and some Plants whom I know nothing about. Since the Faeries have requested them, I know that each of these Plants has a role that they are playing. Sometimes it's obvious: they help to absorb or slow down water, they feed the birds, or they feed pollinators. Sometimes I don't understand their role until years later or possibly never. What I have learned is that the Plants contribute energetically to the Land, helping to create an area for healing and growth. It would be disrespectful of me to ignore the requests of the Nature Spirits and only plant native Plants. This would also inhibit the evolution of the Sanctuary.

I trust that the Nature Spirits and the Plants have a better understanding of what the Land needs than I do, especially for the long run. When an invasive Plant shows up at the Sanctuary, I know that there is a reason. I have heard the argument that invasives are simply good opportunists. Our ecosystems are damaged and so they move in like a grifter looking to take advantage of a bad situation. That's one interpretation. I feel that rather than an opportunist, they are a specialist, like a Red Cross nurse going to a war-torn area, providing the healing that is needed. It is true that they might smother our beloved Plants or native species, but this may also be part of evolution. Or perhaps, the invasive Plant is offering us another opportunity. Unless we work with the invasive Plant, connecting with and listening to ki, we won't know what the Plant's role is. By indiscriminately eradicating ki we miss valuable guidance on what our ecosystem needs.

The word *invasive* comes from *invasion*, which hints toward war or the idea of someone intruding. This furthers the idea of control and dominion over Nature, which, of course, is at the root of our separation. Invasive is limiting, feeding the belief that the world is static, never changing. Invasive allows us to believe that humans know best and that we can determine who belongs and who doesn't. Invasive creates an us (native Plants) versus them (invasive Plants) scenario, feeding the belief of good and bad. We have a war on invasives, eradicating the "bad" Plants who threaten to destroy the economy or the environment (while ignoring the most destructive species currently on Earth). Wouldn't it be a welcome change to stop wasting energy and start working together instead of perpetuating wars? To do so would mean that we might have to acknowledge that humans do not know as much as we think we do and be willing to at least learn from invasives. If we do this, we may just discover that there is no such thing as an invasive Plant.

We have created a false conflict with invasives. However, conflict is an opportunity for connection and growth. When we want what is best for one another (which is best for us), the energetic charge around the conflict disappears. Through reconciliation we engage in Heart-centered creativity to find the best way forward together. This conflict with invasives only exists if we are not in alignment with Nature. Once we decide to be in co-creative partnership with Nature, we realize that we are on the same team. We recognize the gifts of these incredible Plants and understand the role that they are playing in our ecosystem. If we want to save our beloved native Plants, we need to work with the invasives and other Beings of Nature to determine what is needed to bring balance. And we may need to accept that these Beloveds are no longer what is best for this Land. Plants do move around and leave areas; it is part of the natural cycle.

If you continue to struggle with invasives, perhaps you can at least pause and ponder why this war exists in the first place and who bene-fits from labeling Plants as invasive. Or take the time to talk with these Plants to see what they have to say. If we can stop this war on Plants perhaps we can stop the many other wars. After thousands of years, is war really the best that we can do? How much Land have we destroyed, how many people have we killed, how much money have we spent, and how much energy and materials have we wasted in the name of war? And for what? We do not settle conflict through violence. The Plants show us that conflict requires connection. Japanese Hops encourages us to engage.

Taking Action

Here I am finally sitting with Japanese Hops, trying to stay in my Heart while also experiencing feelings of panic over the sensation of an invading army. I take note and push the feeling to the side, trying to see what else is there. As I do, I am mesmerized by the wind blowing over Japanese Hops, resembling waves on an ocean. Slowly I return to calmness and open to the messages of Japanese Hops. Ki points out where ki grows. Hops appeared in several places around the Sanctuary, but the main area where ki grew in absolute abundance was along a drainage culvert that led into the area that was formerly the dump.

By the time I moved to the Sanctuary, I had identified an area where I wanted to work. However, when I sat with the Faeries, they highlighted another area and insisted that this was the first project. As I began to explore this area, I discovered that it was filled with trash. Presumably there had been a burn pile here; however, things piled up and now Plants (primarily Giant Ragweed and Yellow Dock) grew, intermingled with the trash. I had to clear many of the Plants to remove the detritus. Since I was reluctant, it took me almost a year to complete the clean-up. I would start, clear the Plants, remove some junk, get frustrated, and let it go for weeks, only to have to begin again by clearing the Plants that had grown in the interim. I eventually removed the trash and my dad helped me to haul everything to the actual dump. I felt that now that I had finally gotten that job out of the way, I could work on the wetlands, where I had wanted to focus.

A couple weeks after cleaning, we had a deluge. Suddenly the previously dry drainage culvert was overflowing. The water flooded the area that I just cleaned up and then went directly into the creek, carrying with ki the soil, fertilizers, and other poisons from my neighbor's farm. I was stunned, but thought it was a fluke. Before everything could dry, we had more rain, and then more rain, and then more rain. We had so much rain that year that the culvert did not dry out until the following February. (It had been completely dry the first year that I lived here.) It didn't take long for the Faeries to make it clear that this project was not complete.

I realized that I needed to do something to slow the water down and prevent the sediment from flowing into the creek, and that the area of the previous "dump" was important to this project. Beyond that, I had no idea what to do. I left the flooded Sanctuary to teach at a Permaculture Convergence where, serendipitously, I attended a lecture on rain gardens and water catchment. It became clear that I needed to create a rain garden, but this project was even more daunting than the clean-up. First of all, I had no experience with rain gardens. Second, this is a large area. As I continued to work with the Faeries, I began to understand what was needed. We were to create a garden that would help to slow down and soak up the water flowing in from my neighbor's farm, to Plant Bushes and Trees beyond the main garden to help divert the water, and to help prevent the sediment from flowing into the creek. Furthermore, the garden was to shift the energy of the water flowing in so that by the time the molecules got to the creek, they carried the vibration of Love and healing. Together we created the Plant list and a rough design. We planted some of the Bushes and Trees in the surrounding area and that was as far as we got. Despite the guidance, I continued to be overwhelmed with the project. I felt inadequate.

I realized that we needed to create a rain garden in the spring of 2018. Here I am sitting with Japanese Hops in the late summer of 2019, noticing that they are growing along the culvert and the entire rain garden area. As I sat with this Plant, Hops was quick to point out that ki helps to slow down and absorb the water, while also soaking up the excess carbon from the atmosphere and the extra nutrients in the fertilizers from my neighbor's farm. However, ki admonished me for not completing the project that I was asked to do. Hops said that ki was growing there to get my attention and force me to take action. If I did not complete the rain garden, Hops would continue to grow, spreading even further. They gave me permission to clear them from the rain garden.

A couple weeks later, my partner, Marcus, and I started clearing them. The Faeries were adamant that when working in the future rain garden area, we needed to be aware of our emotions. We needed to bring joy and Love to this area. If we were having a bad day or were frustrated or angry, there were other areas where we could work, but we needed to stay out of the rain garden. The energies there were rather precarious and our emotions could greatly affect them. Fortunately, clearing Hops became a fun project. I called it rope wrangling. We had to wear long sleeves and pants because the vines could wrap around us and cause a rash, but other than that it was enjoyable. We soon had enormous piles that towered over our heads. Marcus rolled up an entire area like a giant carpet. As we cleared the Hops, we discovered that they smothered most of the other Plants leaving only Giant Ragweed growing, lessening our work. My teaching assistant, Wendy, joined us and we cleared the whole area rather quickly.

Wendy, my dad, Marcus, and I then built the garden. We call this a rain garden, but it is not a textbook version of one. We did not dig down or put any drainage material underneath. Fortunately, this area naturally created a bowl. We simply spread cardboard, topped this with sticks that were piled in this area, then compost and then planted the garden. It began to rain as Marcus placed the last Plant. We took this as a blessing. This process was a lot of hard work; however, it was completely achievable and it was fun. I needed the push from Japanese Hops to get started. Ki reminded me that we are capable of far more than we realize.

Since then, we have added more Plants to the garden, created a little retention Pond, planted the area around the garden, adding artwork and crystals to support the energy, and planted more surrounding Bushes and Trees, while also shifting our mowed pathways to encourage the water to meander before flowing into the creek. Every year we check in with the rain garden to see if we need to add any other Plants or do any maintenance. Lately we have been expanding the garden to the other side of the culvert. We (mostly Marcus) also remove the Hops from this area and there is less every year. Still, it seems that Hops wants to be sure that we are engaged. We are listening.

One of humanity's gifts is that we are able to move around and create change in our Landscapes. We have mostly abused this gift by creating great harm to Earth. However, if we realign ourselves with Nature and listen to Nature's guidance, we can just as easily utilize this gift to bring healing and beauty to Earth. The Plants are fully aware of our capabilities. They are calling to us, encouraging us to take the actions that are necessary to create a world where all Beings thrive, including humanity.

Time

Japanese Hops wants me to be clear that when I said I didn't have time to sit with ki, I wasn't honest. Yes, I was incredibly busy; however, I created the illusion of no time in order to justify my resistance. In our cultural paradigm, time is linear and finite. There are sixty seconds in a minute, sixty minutes in an hour, twenty-four hours in a day, seven days in a week, and 365 days in a year (plus one more in a leap year). Nature does not adhere to these same rules. Ki recognizes seasons and the movement of time; however, Nature's time is not linear and finite but fluid and flexible. Not every minute contains the same amount of time. When we work with Plants, we discover the expansiveness. I have had experiences where I sat with Plants for what felt like hours and yet, when I came inside, only a few minutes had passed. On a few occasions, I actually gained time.

The Plants also teach us that we can move back and forth in time. Have you ever smelled something and suddenly found yourself back in your grandmother's kitchen (or some other place), experiencing a moment from thirty years ago as if it were right now? This is natural time, often referred to as nonlinear. The Plants help us to go back in time to situations of trauma, as well as situations of Love. Plants also help us to experience the future. They can show us a future place or how a place should look or help us connect with our future self. For instance, when I do Land consultations, the Plants show me something that is meant to be there. It may be a Plant, a piece of artwork, a design, or something else. Sometimes the image is a little vague, but when we find the right component and add this to the Land, I understand what the Plants were suggesting and can feel the vibration of the Land shift. It is more challenging to work in the future because our choices constantly change the possibilities. This is why we cannot determine if humanity will continue living on Earth. We have many choices ahead of us and it is not clear if we will choose to thrive.

Even after all of my years with the Plants, I often think that it is a luxury to spend time with them. They continue to remind me that this is not a luxury but a necessity. Not only does spending time with them help me to be my best self overall, it helps me to be more productive and creative, and gives me insight on how to live in alignment with Nature as well as guidance for myself and my clients. The Plants show me that time is abundant if I allow myself to connect with them.

Importance of Play

Work is prized in our society. Growing up, I often heard someone referred to as a good person because they were a hard worker. They were celebrated for never taking vacations or relaxing. These beliefs are based on capitalism. We are celebrated for being hard workers because we are good cogs in the system, not because this benefits us or Nature.

Japanese Hops reminded us that play is an important part of life for adults just as much as for children, maybe even more so. When we are immersed in the energy of work, often we are fighting against something or engaged in a warring mentality. Play helps us to align with joy and delight—it lightens our energy. Japanese Hops asked us to play. By the end of our day of working with ki, we were sweaty and dirty and tired, but there was much laughter and our Hearts were light. Play gives us permission to experiment and be creative. Imagine if we engaged in all of our work with a sense of play. Maybe our days would be more enjoyable or perhaps we would realize that our work does not serve us.

It might not be feasible to embrace our jobs as play. I'm not sure that I'd like to hear a surgeon say, "Today we're going to play with some knives." But it would be nice that they enjoy their job. The Plants invite us to incorporate play into our lives, to get silly, laugh, and have fun, whenever we can. They say that we humans are too serious. We only live on Earth for a short period of time, and we need to enjoy this incredible gift and delight in the wonders that surround us. Remember, playfulness and joy are positive Heart impulses.

Entering the Daydream of a Plant

Most of our life experiences are from our own perspective. As we mature, we realize that everyone has their own lens, which may be quite different from ours. The beauty of relationships is learning how another experiences the world. When we work with Plants, we realize that they too have a perspective; they experience us as much as we experience them. Entering into the daydream of our Plant ally allows us to sense how they experience the world and gives more insight into who they are.

This is one of my favorite ways of communicating with Plants. From an outside view, it looks like I'm napping with a Plant. I am actually allowing my energy to melt into the Plant. In this process, I feel sensations and a deep sense of gnowing. In this state, I am my Plant ally. I tend to relate to the world kinesthetically, so this experience feels like Home to me. Plus, it gives me an excuse to lie down for a while.

As I daydreamed with Hops, I could feel the energy shift from the invasive army to one of undulating calm. I felt as if I was being rocked by the ocean. I could feel the connections between Hops and the many Beings of Heart Springs Sanctuary, I saw how all are interrelated. I felt Hops pushing me toward the rain garden, both encouraging me and making it very clear what I needed to do.

Exercise: Daydreaming with Your Plant Ally

This is your opportunity to daydream with your Plant ally. During this process, pay close attention to how your body feels. Do you suddenly have any realizations? Feel free to let your imagination run wild. It's fine if you fall asleep.

🖉 You may want to bring a mat or blanket outside to lie on. Place this as close to your Plant ally as possible and lie down. Move into your

Heart space. Feel your body relax, pay attention to your breath as you remember you are breathing in your ally.

🍃 When you are ready, imagine yourself melting into the ground where your Plant ally lives. Your body continues to sink. What sensations do you feel? Allow yourself to merge with the Earth and your Plant. How does your Plant experience this world? How does ki interact with the neighboring Plants?

🍃 Continue to sense and experience your Plant ally.

🍃 When you feel complete, bring your awareness back to your body and your breath. Open your eyes. How does the world appear to you now? How does your body feel?

🍃 Record any observations.

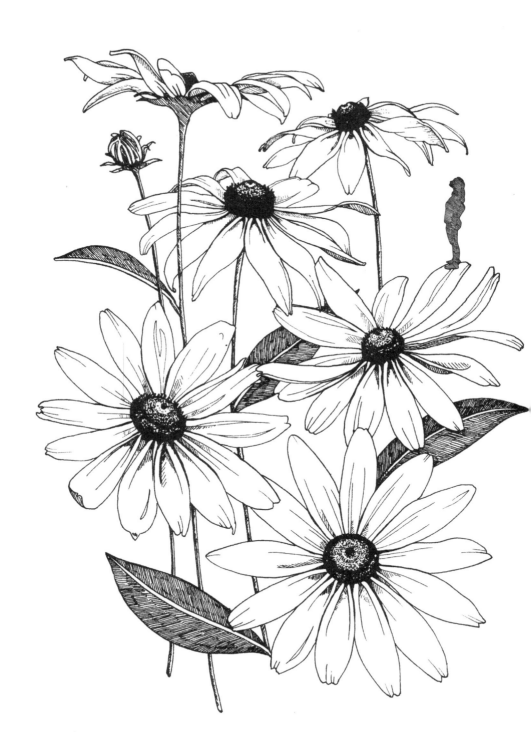

10

❧ Changing Our Story ❧
Black-Eyed Susan

I would like to share a bit of my experience in co-creating this book with the Plants. For about a year, I spent time with the Plants, asking who wanted to be included and what lessons they wanted to share. We compiled a long list and decided to focus on thirty-three Plants. At that time, I was determined to not write a book on Plant communication. As I started writing, I realized that thirty-three Plants was a lot. Either the book would be enormous or I'd only be able to say a few things about each one. I went back to the Plants and the list of lessons and asked if we could combine any. By this point, the Plants made it abundantly clear that they wanted a book about Plant communication, which meant that we had the added layer of the exercises. After months working together, we reduced our list to sixteen Plants, and those are the ones included in this book.

I share this with you to say that I was quite surprised that Black-Eyed Susan (BES) was among the final list of Plants. Don't get me wrong, BES is an incredible Plant whose gifts have changed my life (along with those of my students and clients). Black-Eyed Susan is a special Plant, who I occasionally work with for a very specific reason. But when I talk about light in my classes, I always work with St. John's Wort, one of the foundational Plants of my healing practice and one that is often included in a session or Essence blend. St. John's Wort helps to increase our Soul Force energy, repair the holes in our auras, provide protection, elicit calm, and encourage us to simply be. I feel that almost everyone benefits from regularly working with St. John's Wort.

The main lesson that Black-Eyed Susan shared with me is huge and profound and one that is generally best utilized in a supportive, healing environment. This chapter has been the most challenging for me to write, partially because in order to understand the transformative gift of BES, there needs to be understanding about subconscious patterns, beliefs, and trauma—all subjects that I enjoy but that can make people uncomfortable. I can't even begin to count the number of times that I have questioned the Plants, asking, "Are you sure I shouldn't write about St. John's Wort instead of Black-Eyed Susan?" Truly, St. John's Wort would have been so much easier. But they insist on BES and so I offer you this chapter on changing our story. The irony is not lost on me that a chapter about changing the way in which we experience the world and changing our story has needed to be rewritten so many times that I have lost count.

As a child, I was not a fan of Black-Eyed Susan. It seemed that ki was everywhere, so I took the Plant to be boring. Boy, was I mistaken! At some point, something shifted and I found Black-Eyed Susan to be stunning. I love the juxtaposition of the dark center and bright petals. I too planted ki, and now every year I buy more BES Plants, creating little Black-Eyed Susan communities around the Sanctuary.

While I loved Black-Eyed Susan, I had not worked with ki's Plant Spirit until I assisted Pam Montgomery at a Plant communication weekend in 2015. Prior to attending this weekend, I asked for support or a solution for a couple issues. I wanted a more efficient way to assist my clients in changing their trauma stories and overcoming their limiting beliefs. More personally, I was struggling between wanting to be outside and not wanting to wear sunblock.

As I pulled into the driveway at the retreat center, Black-Eyed Susan (BES) caught my eye. I admired ki's beauty and felt a connection. I was there to support others; I wasn't expecting to spend time with the Plants nor to receive my own healing. However, Black-Eyed Susan captured me and, as I would find out, was able to help me with these very different issues. Once again, Black-Eyed Susan proved that when there is a need, a Plant will emerge to help—we simply need to pay attention and listen.

It's All About Perspective

We have a tendency to believe that the way we experience the world is the only possibility and that the events of our lives are true and fixed. Our perceptions are so vivid that we forget they are merely perceptions, not the full reality. One could ask, what is reality? Our bodies contain more space than matter, yet we perceive them to be solid. They also consist of more bacterial cells than human cells, yet we consider ourselves human and individual rather than recognizing that we are a cooperative community of organisms.

Everything that we experience is based on our perceptions. Everything—the colors we see, the sounds we hear, the flavors we taste, the meaning we give to events—is based on our perceptions, the ways in which our body interprets the signals we receive from the world around us. Black-Eyed Susan says, "It's all about perspective." Ki encourages us to understand that our perceptions inform our experiences.

If we are so fortunate as to meet people from other cultures or people who have different beliefs than us, we may discover that they experience the world quite differently. Within our own family, we witness that we can share the same event and have varying experiences, like my son and I did with the chicken butchering experience I mentioned previously.

Even our memories are not static. Every time we tell a story, the memory is changed, influenced by our current or recent experiences. Sometimes our brain shifts our memories so that they are more in alignment with our beliefs and subconscious patterns, and sometimes they are shifted to protect us—even to the point of complete repression, which is common when one has experienced severe trauma, especially at a young age. Bessel van der Kolk writes, "As long as a memory is inaccessible, the mind is unable to change it. But as soon as a story starts being told, particularly if it is told repeatedly, it changes—the act of telling changes the tale. The mind cannot help but make meaning out of what it knows, and the meaning we make of our lives changes how and what we remember."[1] Black-Eyed Susan informs us that by shifting our perspective, we can shift our experiences and how we interpret them.

The foundation of my healing practice is to help my clients remember who they truly are, which often means clearing away beliefs, behavioral patterns, and energetic blockages that are counter to their Soul, recovering from trauma, and embracing their gifts. As we do this, they look at their lives differently and their story changes.

It is empowering to know that our experiences are not life sentences; we can change our story and the energetic impact of these experiences. There was a time when we did not understand this, when we believed that the events in our lives formed us and there was nothing we could do about it—that we are who we are and nothing could change that. Now we know, however, that our brains are capable of changing more than we thought possible, even to the point of creating new brain cells and neural pathways. Black-Eyed Susan reminds us that what we think is true is only part of the story. Ki invites us to take another look with a different perspective. By doing so, we come to know the truth of who we are.

When discussing perspectives, I often think about flipping through the different lenses at the eye doctor's office as the doctor asks, "Which lens is better?" We have an understanding that lenses affect the way in which we see the world; whether they are magnifying, wide-angled, or tinted, we can swap them out and see the world differently. We each have many layers of lenses that affect our perceptions, all of which are changeable. The lenses with the greatest impacts are those of our subconscious patterns, beliefs, traumas (including those inherited from our Ancestors), and momentous experiences.

Subconscious Patterns

According to Bruce Lipton, our subconscious mind is in "control" about 95 percent of the time.[2] Thank goodness! Our bodies need to process tens of millions of stimuli every second. We would go crazy if we had to consciously process and respond to each stimulus. To efficiently process an enormous amount of information, the subconscious mind relies on patterns based on previous experiences. The more we have experienced a particular pattern, the more ingrained it is. This efficiency, however, makes it difficult to approach experiences with innocent perception.

The foundation for these patterns formed during our early childhood years, as we observed our parents, caregivers, environment, and community. If you watch young children, they are both sponges and mirrors, soaking up the world around them and reflecting it back to us. They are incredibly sensitive and more open to energetics and emotions than most adults. Children are dependent on others for their basic needs; therefore, this sensitivity is a survival mechanism to help them learn how to navigate the world and thrive. As they witness the interactions around them, they begin to assign meaning to them. If a parent screams whenever they see a spider, the child thinks, "Spiders are scary." If their parent gives them attention or praises them whenever they bring their parent a Dandelion they think, "Flowers and gifts are good." This is an oversimplification, but basically, we are domesticated by our parents and caregivers during our early years through the messages we receive from them. We want to survive, we want to thrive, we want Love, and therefore our subconscious determines the patterns that are most likely to get us what we want.

Fortunately our subconscious patterns are changeable. Sometimes the shift is simply making a choice to respond differently. Other times it may take considerable effort, but we are able to shift these patterns so that they are more in alignment with how we want to experience the world or who we are. For example, a child who was taught to take care of others or who learned to read their volatile parent's needs to avoid eruptions may, as an adult, find themselves taking care of everyone else while neglecting themselves. This pattern often results in exhaustion, depletion, and illness, which is their body's way of forcing them to take a break and pay attention to their own needs—their illness is an invitation to shift their pattern of putting others before themselves. They may simply need to make a choice to put themselves first. Or they may need to do more healing work, focusing on shifting the pattern and underlying beliefs and traumas. Shifting this pattern will affect their perspective and how they experience the world, as well as help them to live a more Soul-aligned life.

Beliefs

As we grow and learn, our beliefs are meant to change, especially when we are presented with new information. I like to think of beliefs as costumes or different-colored sunglasses. We put them on and get to see what the world is like from this perspective. Perhaps it feels right until we do a costume change and suddenly we realize that the previous costume didn't fit as well as the new one—in comparison it feels restrictive and outdated. Ideally, our beliefs become more expansive and inclusive, incorporating more of the possibilities of life. We call this being openminded; it manifests in having a more fluid and substantial mental body, which allows us to have a wider perspective.

Unfortunately, beliefs have become an identifier. We use them to describe ourselves and to form our associations or to explain our othering. When we define who we are based on our beliefs, we become rigid and locked in a box, our mental body becoming thin and hard, rendering us unable to connect with people who have differing beliefs. We limit our experience of the world and we make it difficult to change our perspective, thus reducing our chances of healing and growing.

While we are engaged in our healing work, it is helpful to be mindful of our beliefs, especially those that seem to be counter to who we are. Like our subconscious patterns, many of our beliefs are formed during our early childhood years or are inherited from our family, Ancestors, and culture. We want to weed out any beliefs that are interfering with following our Soul Path and being who we are meant to be.

Sometimes we try to shift our subconscious patterns and beliefs with affirmations. Affirmations are wonderful but since they focus on the conscious mind, if they are not accompanied with action or changed behavior they are rarely effective. It does not matter how beautiful our words are or how many self-help books we can quote; if they are not in alignment with our beliefs and subconscious patterns, they have little effect on us. Affirmations can also backfire as we blame ourselves, wondering why they are not working or why they aren't true for us. Focusing on them may create a superficial change but not address the underlying story. If we want affirmations to be true in our core, we need to focus on the underlying issues—such as our beliefs, patterns, and traumas. That being said, affirmations can be helpful to reframe and shift course when we are addressing subconscious or habitual behavior patterns, or when we find ourselves falling back into an old pattern we thought we had left behind. We can pause, recognize that this is an old pattern, and state the new pattern we are creating. For example, when we make a mistake, we might find ourselves falling into an old pattern of belittling ourselves by saying, "Why can't I do anything right? Everyone else has it together. I'm such a loser." When this occurs, we want to pause, breathe, and recognize that these statements are part of an old subconscious pattern, and we are no longer following that path. We may then want to remind ourselves of the new pattern using affirmations: "It's okay to make mistakes. I'm only human. This is a learning opportunity. I can make mistakes and be a good person who is worthy of Love." To help strengthen this shift, we want to do something that embraces mistakes or self-acceptance. I once knitted a challenging (for me) scarf and didn't allow myself to pull out any of my mistakes. In the end, I thought the mistakes were the parts that added the most beauty. Again, working with affirmations needs to include action and changed behavior, not just beautiful words, to successfully shift our subconscious patterns and beliefs.

Trauma

The more that I questioned writing about Black-Eyed Susan and trauma, the more the Plants insisted. Yes, Black-Eyed Susan's gifts are incredible and understanding the impacts of trauma on our perspective is helpful, but the Plants want to stress that as we go through trauma (from the original experience to the suppression to the recovery), the Plants are there to support us. They say, "You are never alone. You are Love(d) as you are." No matter how traumatized we are, the Plants are there to remind us of our innate Sacredness and to guide us back to our Soul Path.

The word *trauma* is tossed about frequently. It can be a charged term, and often elicits judgment and fear. Trauma is an inherent part of our life. When we discuss trauma, there is a common response of discounting our experiences or thinking, "Others had it worse than me," or not understanding why someone considers an event traumatic. What we define as traumatic largely depends on our previous life experiences and beliefs. There is no point in comparing the severity of trauma; it is all relative and we have all experienced trauma. We can try to avoid it, suppress it, and dissociate from it, but these attempts only compound the trauma. In essence, it is not the event that matters, but the story that is connected to it, how our body responds to this story, and how we define ourselves based on our interpretation of the story or the meaning we have assigned to it. When we address our trauma, we empower ourselves to truly heal and change our lives.

Our understanding of trauma and its impacts has deepened considerably in recent years. I find these new discoveries and understandings to be incredibly exciting because they enable us to more fully heal and recover from trauma, and they help to remove the old stigma around trauma and therapy. In addition, we are discovering that much of what we thought was intrinsic to our personalities or even our culture is actually a response to trauma. Trauma specialist, Resmaa Menakem says, "Trauma decontextualized in a person looks like personality. Trauma decontextualized in a family looks like family traits. Trauma in a people looks like culture."[3] Ultimately, these discoveries mean that we have more control over our lives than we thought and by healing our traumas (individual and collective), we can create a more loving world that honors all of life.

Trauma and recovery from trauma are enormous, multilayered subjects that reach far beyond the scope of this book. Our focus here is the relationship between trauma and our perspective. Like looking through a fish-eye lens, trauma, especially childhood trauma, distorts our perspective. Trauma also influences our subconscious patterns and beliefs. We experience a physiological response to trauma, which can alter our brain functionality and the way in which we experience the world. In his incredible book *The Body Keeps the Score,* Bessel van der Kolk writes:

> . . . trauma is not just an event that took place sometime in the past; it is also the imprint left by that experience on mind, brain, and body. This imprint has ongoing consequences for how the human organism manages to survive in the present.
>
> Trauma results in a fundamental reorganization of the way mind and brain manage perceptions. It changes not only how we think and what we think about, but also our very capacity to think.[4]

As the title of van der Kolk's book suggests, the imprint of trauma resides in our body even when we do not have a memory or understanding of it.

Trauma keeps us locked in the past. We can be going about our lives when we encounter a trigger and suddenly our world shifts. Our bodies respond as if we are experiencing the original trauma—remember, time is not linear. We are no longer in our rational brain nor in our Heart space; rather, we are responding from survival mode. In these moments, we are facing a very different scenario than what everyone else around us is experiencing, which can be frightening to all involved. Often, we do not have a recollection of the actual event or possibly even what triggered us. We simply start to feel emotions, commonly fear or anger, which may result in a panic attack or other physical symptoms.

When we are triggered, it is helpful to bring our attention to our bodies and our immediate surroundings. I like to ask, "What are my hands doing? Where are my feet?" Sometimes we have to do this again and again until we can become aware of our present moment. Focusing on our breathing (breathing in through the nose and out through the mouth, as slowly as possible) while reminding ourselves that we are safe is also helpful. Spending time in Nature, especially with a Tree or beloved Plant, can help us to calm and return to our bodies and the present moment. Pete Walker has a valuable list of thirteen steps for managing flashbacks in his book, *Complex PTSD: From Surviving to Thriving.*[5] Being triggered signals that we have unprocessed traumas and encourages us to do the work necessary to heal the wounds. We take the sting out of the triggers when we recognize the opportunity that they present.

As we look over our life events and traumas, it is helpful to remember that by nature we are resilient. Research shows that if we have someone who is genuinely interested in our well-being, comforts us, and loves us, we are generally able to recover from horrible experiences relatively unscathed. But if we do not have this support or, worse, if the people who are meant to care for us are the ones who inflict trauma on us, we are less resilient, and our experiences can have disastrous impacts. The monumental Adverse Childhood Experiences (ACE) Study demonstrates that child abuse has long-lasting, potentially life-long consequences, including greater incidence of disease, alcoholism, incarceration, drug abuse, suicide, depression, domestic violence, and learning and behavioral problems. Robert Anda, one of the investigators of the study, concluded ". . . that they had stumbled upon the gravest and most costly public health issue in the United States: child abuse."[6] Often when we think of child abuse, we think of extreme physical or sexual violence; however, there are a wide range of experiences that constitute child abuse including verbal insults, belittling or shaming, contempt, abandonment, emotional and physical neglect, rage, adults not honoring the Soul growth of the child, and witnessing other family members being harmed.

The effects of child abuse are long-lasting in part due to the changes trauma causes in the child's developing brain. Bessel van der Kolk explains, "If you feel safe and loved, your brain becomes specialized in exploration, play, and cooperation; if you are frightened and unwanted, it specializes in managing feelings of fear and abandonment."[7] Trauma, especially repeated trauma, often results in hypersensitivity and hypervigilance, where we are always on alert, believing that the world is unsafe, possibly interpreting benign experiences as dangerous. In other words, the lens of trauma has distorted our perspective. Taken to the extreme, we may find it difficult to function as part of society and may feel unsafe whenever we are around others. Traumatic experiences can greatly interfere with our experience of the world and our sense of self. The hypervigilance of always being on alert prevents our bodies from moving into restorative mode, interfering with our health and growth.

The discoveries of the ACE Study encourage us to look at our childhood experiences in a new way. We are able to let go of the shame and blame and embrace compassion when, for example, we can see that we weren't "bad" kids; we were simply kids who developed responses to a bad situation. Even more importantly, it becomes easier to know ourselves and to find our way to healing. The findings also encourage us to shift our society to enable happier, healthier children.

Trauma does not just include the events that we experienced or personally witnessed. We can be traumatized by communal events, such as a school shooting, the 9/11 attacks, or species collapse. Epigenetics shows us that trauma (along with fears and beliefs) can be passed down to future generations through changes in gene expression. The egg that formed you was formed inside your mother while your grandmother was pregnant with her. While I love the poetry of this, it demonstrates how we can be affected by events that occurred long before we were born. The stresses, beliefs, and life events that your grandmother experienced before giving birth to your mother can affect your own health and well-being. Your grandmother was once an egg inside your great-great grandmother's body. It becomes easy to see how trauma is compounded through generations, meaning that we are affected by experiences that are far removed from our present lives.

If we look back over the history of humanity, we see that we have inherited a long history of trauma. Many of the atrocities that have occurred were expressions of unhealed trauma, which only compounded the pain and continued a cycle of trauma. This understanding invites us to look at world events with a different perspective. For example, we can see that the colonists who came to North America were fleeing centuries of persecution focused on separating their innate connection with Nature and the Divine. They attempted to deflect this pain onto the Land, the Indigenous people who were here, and the people who were kidnapped and sold into slavery. In doing so, they followed the long-held pattern of oppressed people becoming oppressors.

While it may be overwhelming to think about all the traumatic events that have occurred throughout human history, in our families, or in our own lives, it gives me hope because the key here is unhealed trauma. Unhealed trauma makes a prisoner out of us, keeping us from experiencing our fullness. And worse, the coping mechanisms and reactions from our unhealed trauma radiate out, often causing harm to others while contributing to our own dis-ease.

We no longer need to be defined by these traumatic experiences. Black-Eyed Susan encourages us to look at them with a different perspective, reminding us that we absolutely can shift their energetic imprint and the meanings that we attach to them—meaning that we can heal and recover from trauma. When we do, we impact others, helping the healing to ripple out. While this can be a painful process (it can also be an enjoyable experience), in the long run, healing our trauma saves us an enormous amount of anguish and helps us to have a healthier and more enjoyable life. I have witnessed relatively fast recovery from traumas, and sometimes the healing process is long and circuitous. There are many modalities that help to heal trauma. In the end, the best modality is the one that works for you.

Remember, our bodies are incredibly resilient. It's also important to note that sometimes trauma can have a positive effect; realizing its impact can help us become softer, more compassionate, more loving, or help us learn the lessons we need including to speak up for ourselves or set boundaries. A traumatic event can sometimes cause us to reevaluate and reprioritize our lives. As we heal, we are more able to recognize the potential gifts and learning opportunities of these experiences.

Changing Our Story

As we investigate our perspective, we discover that the lenses that form it are mostly subconscious. The formation of our perspective is based on the conscious and unconscious messages and values communicated to us from before birth, resulting in a perspective that has been greatly influenced by other people during a time when we did not have much conscious control over our lives. This means that our interpretation of the world, our health, and even our life story is substantially created by others. Since our experiences are based on our perceptions, we can change how we experience the world and, ultimately, our life's story. If we want to know who we truly are and create a life aligned with our Soul, we want to shift our lens. Doing so not only offers us a different perspective, but releases us from the burdens and limitations we have (mostly unknowingly) been carrying and changes the energetic imprints held by our bodies, potentially altering our health and genetic expression, as well as those of our descendants.

Changing our story in this manner is embodied; it is not merely editing to ignore or remove the parts that we don't like. When we change our story, we take ownership of our life, becoming the author. In order to do so, we need to have a willingness to change and to consider other possibilities. As our story changes, we may discover that other aspects of our lives also change, including our relationships, because we are no longer acting out of our trauma responses and limiting beliefs (or at least we do so less often). We have a better understanding of ourselves and are able to live a more authentic, conscious, and Soul-aligned life. Black-Eyed Susan helps us to shed false narratives, embrace who we are, and stand in our radiant truth.

I have focused on the three most common categories of lenses that have the biggest negative impact on our perspective (beliefs, patterns, and traumas). It is important to mention that our perspective is also influenced through positive experiences. Ask any loving parent and they will tell you that having a child affected the way in which they see the world. Moments of connection, awe, Love, pleasure, and contentment can inform our perspective. They can also help to heal trauma and shift our subconscious patterns and beliefs.

Sometimes the best thing that we can do for ourselves, our descendants, and our world is to seek out these enjoyable moments that make life more beautiful and meaningful. These moments can be momentous or mundane. If they are nourishing our Heart and Soul, they are influencing our perspective. This is especially important if your experiences or traumas have impacted your ability to feel safe in the world.

Embracing Perfectly Imperfect

The common belief that one is bad or toxic interferes with our healing. People with this belief were frequently made to believe that something was wrong with them or that they didn't fit in as they were growing up. The belief manifests in several ways. One is constantly forcing oneself to dive deep to "heal" the hidden or wounded aspects, thinking that if we can heal these "less desirable" aspects of ourselves then we will no longer be bad or toxic. This approach assumes that healing is hierarchical, that we can progress in a linear fashion and arrive at a certain level if we only do enough healing. The problem is that there is no end destination. We continually evolve. As I tell my clients, if you are alive, then there is healing work to do. But that does not mean that we need to be constantly looking for pain and drama. Our wounds and growth opportunities present themselves when we are ready to heal. We don't have to go searching. (Being curious about why something is happening in your life or why you believe something is not the same as continually diving deep.) The deep dive can act like a drug and a distraction. It can also be traumatizing. Constantly digging is like looking for a splinter that isn't there. We start digging, and when we don't find something, we go deeper and deeper, until we are feeling raw. Now we have an infected wound that needs attention. Had we not gone searching, the wound would not have occurred.

Another way that the belief that we are bad or toxic manifests is when we interpret the presentation of a lesson or healing opportunity as confirmation that we are bad or wrong. We think, "I already addressed this. Why is this coming up again? Did I do something wrong?" Again, healing is not linear; it is commonly referred to as a spiral, and there are usually many layers to our healing. One of my main lessons in life is the importance of patience. I cannot even begin to count the number of times that I needed to learn this lesson or experience a healing connected to it. Again, there is no destination; we cannot slide back nor can we leap forward. If a healing or growth opportunity is presenting itself again, then it is simply a sign that we have an opportunity for healing.

We are not wrong or bad or toxic. We have wounds and lessons.

Yes, we all have healing work to do *and* we are perfect as we are; as a friend says, we are "perfectly imperfect." Like a Plant blooming, we can heal and grow into our next evolution. But this is not a constant process. Everything in life rests. Black-Eyed Susan does not bloom all year long—ki does not even bloom all summer long. Ki needs to take a rest, focus on other aspects of life. We too need to rest and to enjoy and appreciate life, remembering all that is going well, both personally and in the world. It is these moments that bring meaning to life and give us the energy and momentum to continue with the work of healing. We do not benefit from the continual deep dive. Since Love is the most powerful healer there is, we can just as easily heal and grow through Love and pleasure. When we need a reminder, Black-Eyed Susan is there to tell us that we are perfect and loved just as we are.

Receiving the Gifts of Black-Eyed Susan

Helping people change their stories, shift their beliefs and habitual patterns, and embrace their truth is a large part of my healing practice. I have a number of tools and practices as well as Plant allies who assist in this process. However, before meeting the Spirit of Black-Eyed Susan, I was looking for a way to make this process more efficient and effective. During a Plant communication class, I asked my guides if there was a modality I should study or a Plant who could help. As I waited for a response, I became observant. Of course, Black-Eyed Susan became the answer. While BES's gift of changing perspectives is abundantly clear to me now, it was not obvious from the beginning, so I will explain how I came to this realization.

First, I made the request. This is an important step that I continually stress to my students and clients: ask the Plants for what you need. Then Black-Eyed Susan caught my attention. At this point, I hadn't even considered that BES was the answer I was looking for, but it was clear that ki wanted to connect and be in relationship. As I sat with BES, I noticed that my perspective was shifting. Sounds distorted. My vision was changing. I (fully awake) saw Black-Eyed Susan towering over me as I climbed up ki's stem. Colors and light changed. While journeying with ki (see chapter 13), my perspectives continued to shift. As I sat with BES again, I was encouraged to experience ki from different angles and distances, and each one presented a new perspective. Then, I received the message from Black-Eyed Susan: "I can help your clients find a different perspective for their stories." As we continued to talk, Black-Eyed Susan told me that ki helps "change people's stories." I realized that Black-Eyed Susan was the answer to my request.

After the Plant communication class ended, I continued to work with Black-Eyed Susan to discover how ki helped change people's stories. Black-Eyed Susan taught me that, "It's all about the perspective and the lens through which we see the world." Ki helps to shift our perspective, which "changes the meaning and energetic imprints of the events in our lives." As I played with Black-Eyed Susan, BES showed me how to work with ki to shift perspectives. I experimented with this and saw how Black-Eyed Susan helped me to look at past traumas or an issue in a new way, which then caused me to shift the story that I assigned to them. Later, I shared this process with my students and a few clients and discovered that they had similar experiences. I now had enough confirmation to say confidently that Black-Eyed Susan helps us to overcome trauma, shift our beliefs, and rewrite our stories by changing the way in which we see the world.

While Black-Eyed Susan was shifting my perspective during the class, I also noticed that I was sitting in the intense mid-day sun without getting burned. Since many sunscreens contain chemicals that are known carcinogens, I prefer to use them sparingly. However, I have extremely fair skin—the running joke is that the only way I tan is when my freckles connect. I usually can only be in the sun for about twenty minutes before burning, which interferes with my work at the Sanctuary. Knowing that the Plants are able to convert Sunlight, I turned to them and asked who could help me absorb more sunlight. I wondered if Black-Eyed Susan was my answer again. After working with BES, I was able to increase my time in the sun to several hours before burning. But I also learned that there is a limit to this protection that must be respected.

One day as I was weeding the Strawberry patch, I kept receiving the message that the time was up—I needed to go inside. I wanted to finish the project and kept asking Black-Eyed Susan to help me absorb the sun and continued working for about another hour, and I received a severe sunburn. Since that day, I know when I'm told that the time is up, I need to go inside or at least put on sunscreen. Still, I am grateful to Black-Eyed Susan for helping me to absorb more sunlight without getting burned.

Judgment

Sitting with Black-Eyed Susan, I felt a tingling in my crown chakra. At the time this did not make sense to me and I ignored it, which only made the sensation more pronounced. After several sittings, I looked at Black-Eyed Susan with a loupe and saw that the center was not black as I had assumed but purple, the color associated with the crown chakra. As I continued to connect with Black-Eyed Susan, ki reminded me of the danger of judgment. Again, judgment closes the Heart and limits our experiences. Judgment clouds our lens. If we express judgment toward another Being, we dismiss their value and wholeness and create a separation.

We want to engage in innocent perception, meeting each experience without preconceived notions. I know this, I teach this, and yet here I was, not utilizing this important skill. We all stumble at times; the key is to recognize it and try again.

Curiosity is an antidote to judgment. When we experience something that doesn't quite make sense to us, we can pause and get curious. Curiosity encourages us to look at different perspectives, to ask questions and discover more information. Curiosity opens the door to other possibilities. Remember—our brains want to create coherence with our patterns and past experiences, and curiosity creates a pause, providing us with the potential to move beyond these patterns. When we engage with respectful curiosity, we promote communion as well as compassion and understanding, which results in Heart coherence.

We benefit from employing more curiosity in our interactions with one another. When we are confronted with someone who has beliefs that differ from ours, we are often quick to judge them—they are uneducated, they are too politically correct, they are delusional—so that we can dismiss them. If we remember the lessons of Black-Eyed Susan, we can perhaps take a different approach, engaging with curiosity, shifting our perspective, and perhaps creating a new story. Even if we cannot accept the perspective that this Being presents, we may be able to have some understanding.

Light

Light is a powerful phenomenon. Think of all the ways in which light is mentioned. "Walk toward the light." "In the beginning there was light." Anyone associated with natural healing has heard, "Sending you Love and light" or "Imagine healing light pouring into you."

In the electrified world, it is easy to take light for granted. And yet, can you imagine a world without light? Life as we know it, if it could even exist, would be very different. Light is integral to life. We need light for our health; sunlight helps in the creation of Vitamin D, which is important for strong bones and teeth as well as a healthy immune system. Light also greatly affects our emotional well-being, as evidenced by Seasonal Affective Disorder (SAD).

We contain light at the core of our being, in each of our cells. Or, as German physicist Fritz-Albert Popp says, "We know today that man, essentially, is a being of light."[8] In 1970, expanding on the experiments of Russian biologist Alexander Gurwitsch, Popp proved the existence of biophotons, particles of ultra-weak light with no mass, that transmit information between and within the cell. Biophotons have been shown to exist in the nucleus of the cells in almost all biological species, including humans. What's more, Popp and his successors have demonstrated that healthy cells emit a different frequency of light than diseased cells. Popp in particular focused on cancer cells, discovering that cancer acts like a light scrambler causing the light emitted by cells to become less coherent.[9]

Popp's discoveries show that in addition to potentially providing benefits to our health, biophotons are a primary form of communication within and among living organisms. In other words, our bodies utilize light to share information both internally and with the outer world. As we move through the world, sharing our messages of light, our more-than-human relatives respond in kind. It appears as if light is the universal language. Who better to guide our relationship with light than Plants? After all, Plants transform sunlight into food or usable energy, which in turn becomes food for others. Plants act as light translators for us. It only makes sense that working with Plants can improve our health as they can affect the frequency of our biophotons.

Sometimes the importance of light gets mistranslated into the idea of light and dark as good and bad, respectively. We need to be cautious of this belief and notice when it occurs, for it is rooted in racism. Light is important and healing. So is darkness. Cultures around the world utilize darkness either by going into a cave, blindfolding, or using another form of light deprivation to promote visualization, healing, and receiving guidance. The dark is where we plant our seeds. We ourselves are formed in the dark. Life requires both light and dark; both are vital, both are beautiful, and both are magical.

Color

Much of our experience with light is through the form of color. There is a tendency to make a cursory observation of a Plant's color, similar to what I originally did with Black-Eyed Susan. Remember, our brains like patterns. When we look at a lawn, our brains tell us that it is green. But if we take the time to look closer, we find a multitude of shades of green plus many other colors such as red, brown, and yellow. We can use innocent perception to regularly notice the varied colors of our surroundings.

Color is a language that can provide clues to a Plant's gifts. This language is multilayered, affecting us on different levels including emotionally, energetically, and physically. While there are guidelines to the meaning and effects of color, ultimately, this is a personal experience. We each resonate more with particular colors, which can change depending on the day, time of day, season, or our mood.

Light travels in waves and the distance between these waves is called a wavelength. Most humans can only see a small part of the spectrum of light known as visible light. Our eyes perceive the different wavelengths of visible light as having different colors. This is because our eyes have three types of photoreceptor cells called cones. Each is able to sense a different range of wavelengths. We refer to these cones as long-wavelength sensitive (L), which sense the red spectrum; medium-wavelength sensitive (M), which sense the green spectrum; and short-wavelength sensitive (S), which sense the blue spectrum. With these three types of cones, we are able to perceive millions of unique colors.

Once again, color is perceived. When someone only has two types of cones or has a low functioning third type of cone, we refer to them as "color blind." They do not see as wide of a range of colors as the average person. This adaptation also makes it challenging for them to see contrast. Some people (referred to as tetrachromats) have four types of cones—this allows them to see up to 100 million colors! We are also learning that animals have varying visual systems. Bees, butterflies, and many birds and animals are able to see ultraviolet light. Photographing Plants and animals under ultraviolet light reveals patterns that are not apparent in the visible light spectrum. Apparently, beauty is in the eye of the beholder, and dependent on what the beholder can see. Ultimately, color is about the relationship between the observer and the observed.

Besides the personal experience of color, there are color correspondences, which I consider to be guidelines or clues more than hard and fast rules. Color correspondences can be culture dependent. For instance, when I work with Rocío Alarcón, we consider red to be protective. While in Damanhur, black is protective.

There are correspondences between colors and the chakras. Chakras are energy centers—sometimes referred to as energetic organs—in our bodies that spiral out through our auras. *Chakra* is a Sanskrit word meaning "wheel." While chakras have been widely incorporated into Western culture, we continue to learn about them and their importance in our lives. Red is associated with the root chakra, which is located at the base of our spine and is connected to feeling safe, grounded, and in our bodies. Orange is associated with the second or hara chakra, which is at the place of the womb or between the tail bone and belly button. This chakra is connected to fertility (of all forms) and sexuality, as well as desire, pleasure, boundaries, creativity, and how we engage with others. The solar plexus chakra is located at your belly and has to do with self-esteem, finances, how we present ourselves to the world, our force of will, our relationship to power, and our sense of self. I think of this chakra as your shining star. Yellow is considered to be the color for this chakra. Are you seeing a pattern?

The fourth chakra is our Heart chakra, which of course is connected to Love and being Love(d). This chakra is the mid-point, uniting the Above and Below. This is the place of universal connection, compassion, and forgiveness. Two colors are associated with the Heart chakra: green and pink. Plants predominantly emit the color that resonates with our Heart chakra; they are bathing us with Love. Blue is the color connected to our fifth chakra, our throat chakra. This chakra is concerned with speaking our truth, being heard, and how we express ourselves, including creatively. Our sixth chakra is the first eye chakra. Many refer to the first eye as the third eye. I heard Margi Flint refer to this chakra as the first eye chakra and have referred to the chakra by this name ever since. This is the place of our intuition, where we see clearly, visualize, and gnow. I want my intuition to be my primary sight; therefore, this is my *first* eye. This chakra is associated with the color indigo. Our seventh chakra is our crown chakra, located at the top of our head and extending upward. This is the place where we connect to the Divine, the universe, and consciousness. Violet (and sometimes white) is the color associated with the crown chakra. This is a very simplified description of our chakras; however, it provides a clue for the possible gifts of our Plants.

Not every Plant is associated with a chakra. However, if they are, they can help us to balance or keep that chakra vibrant. For example, Dandelion is a great third chakra Plant with ki's radiant yellow, helping us to shine brightly, and Blue Borage strengthens our throat chakra, giving us courage to speak our truth.

There are also color correspondences to parts of our bodies. For instance, yellow is connected to bile, our liver, and gallbladder. Red has a relationship with our blood. White is often considered to be connected to our bones and sometimes the nervous system. Indigo is associated with pain relief. Again, these are possible associations, not definite connections.

We associate emotions with certain colors. Common correlations are red and anger; blue and sadness; yellow and happiness; green and envy; or black and depression, grief, and death. These associations are greatly affected by cultural beliefs and one's own personality. I do not like to wear black; I feel my energy gets depleted when I wear this color. I have friends whose wardrobe almost entirely consists of black. This color uplifts and comforts them.

While our experience of color may be subjective, it is an energetic exchange that has the ability to provide information and insights. Plus it can be a lot of fun to immerse oneself in the colors of your Plant. When engaging with the color of your Plant, try to resist preconceived notions. Allow yourself to be filled with this color and notice your experiences.

Exercise: Engaging with Color with Your Plant Ally

🌿 Using innocent perception, observe the entirety of your Plant. If ki is large, you may need to stand some distance away to take in the full view of your Plant. What is the color that first captures your attention? What is the overall expression of color? Do you feel this somewhere in your body? Does this elicit any sensations or memories?

🌿 Close your eyes and connect with your Plant friend. Is there a color that comes to mind as you connect with ki?

🌿 Focus on the details. Look closely at the different parts of your Plant. What colors are on the stem, leaves, petals? It is helpful to use a loupe or magnifying glass to get a close look. If your Plant has flowers, be sure to look at the pollen. What other colors are present or hidden? For some Plants, an important color is in their roots, like Bloodroot or Goldenseal. If it is possible to do so without harming your Plant, look at ki's roots or look at a picture of your Plant's roots.

🍂 What sensations do these colors provoke? How does your body feel as you absorb these colors? What messages or stories do the colors share with you? You may wish to journal about your impressions, or even paint a picture once you have absorbed the experience.

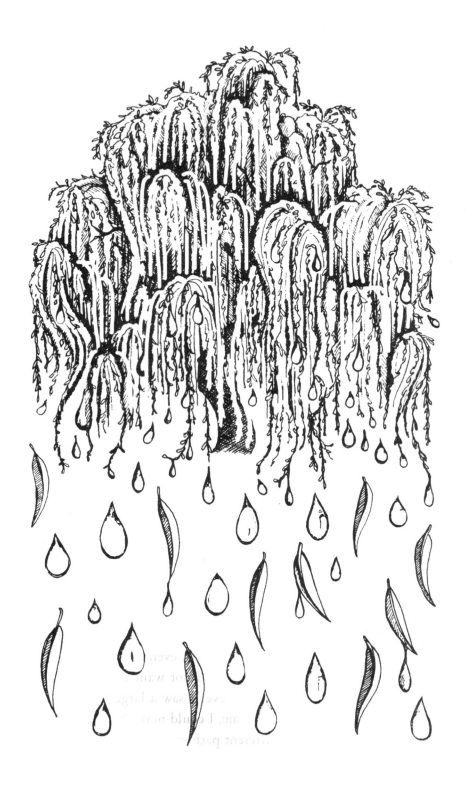

11
❧ Releasing Grief ❧
Willow

*I*s there a more romantic Tree than Willow? Weeping Willow begs you to lie down, have a picnic, or go for a swing, forgetting all your troubles and simply enjoying the pleasure of life. I have long loved Weeping Willows; my Heart would light up at the sight of one across a field. My relationship with Willow shifted surprisingly years ago when I participated in a class led by Starhawk. We were asked to go outside, close our eyes, and allow ourselves to be drawn to a Plant, and then experience this Plant with our other senses. I was drawn to Willow. I remember caressing ki's branches and leaves. My Heart kept opening further and further as my body relaxed. I could feel energy building between us. I felt deeply connected and an enormous Love for this Tree. The energy continued to increase to the point that I experienced an orgasm and shifted into a state of Divine bliss.

I was astonishingly shocked. I never had an experience like this. There I was, standing at a local college, completely clothed, surrounded by a large group of people, having an orgasm with a Willow Tree! I did not know how to process this or even how to explain what happened, which was fine because I did not want to talk to anyone about it. For years afterward, whenever I saw a large Willow Tree I would blush. While this shocked me, I could never have guessed how this would lead me down a different path many years later.

We all have defining moments in our life, those moments that divide our lives into "before" and "after." We have these collectively, such as 9/11 and COVID, and we also have our personal measurements. Probably the most defining moment for me occurred in 2011. While this moment was incredibly painful, it also greatly shifted my life, resulting in an absurd amount of beauty and pleasure.

The summer after experiencing my life changing event, I lost all of my resistance. I no longer had the energy for it. I barely had energy for anything. This is how I found myself sitting in a class with Pam Montgomery at the New England Women's Herbal Conference. I remember Pam was talking about the Heart and Heart intelligence. She was beaming because she just recently married her Beloved, Mark. Pam mentioned a transformative experience of orgasming with White Pine. I couldn't believe it! By this point, I studied with and read many books by amazing Plant people and yet I never heard anyone else mention an experience like I had had with Willow. That is when I knew that I needed to learn more from Pam. (She briefly shares her experience with White Pine in her book *Plant Spirit Healing*.[1])

Sacred Sex

Since that time, I have studied Sacred sex and am able to understand my experience with Willow. Our Western culture has a skewed (and unhealthy) view of sex and sexuality, which has resulted in rape culture, sexual dysfunctions, unnecessary shame, and too many people experiencing unsatisfactory sex (even when they don't realize it). Sacred sex is healing and empowering for ourselves and the greater whole. When we recognize the possibilities that can occur through Sacred sex, including magic and power, we understand why some institutions try to control, demonize, and limit our sexual experiences. As Pam Montgomery writes, "Perhaps part of our evolution is taking the erotic out of the realm of debasement and bringing it into the realm of the sacred."[2]

At the core, sex is an energetic exchange that leads to union, connection, and ideally the creation of Love. We absolutely can have this exchange without penetration. We have these amazing, glorious bodies who are capable of experiencing and giving pleasure in bountiful ways. Why would we want to limit this? When you understand how to move energy and how to connect with someone else's energy (be they another human, Willow, or rock), you can experience an orgasm any time, anywhere. Sacred sex teaches us, however, that orgasm is not the end goal, but only a potential opening for increasing the energy; the true goal is union. We utilize the energy created through our union to tap into Unity Consciousness, experience the Divine, receive healing, or benefit the world in another way. (There is a difference between orgasm and ejaculation. It can be a challenge for people with a penis to separate the two. When they learn this technique, a whole new world opens up for both them and their partners. It's well worth the effort to learn how to separate orgasm from ejaculation.)

We sometimes refer to sex as making Love, which conjures images of sweetness and softness that some call boring. Actually, making Love does just that—it makes (or creates) Love. When engaged in Sacred sex, we have the capacity to create the energy of Love, increasing the amount of Love in this world. How incredible! If you are frustrated by the state of the world, if you are overwhelmed by hate, you can shift this and bring healing by making Love. There is good reason why the Beltane ceremonies include blessing the Land with ceremonial sex. The energy that is created through the alchemical process of Sacred sex can be utilized for healing ourselves, the Land, the world, and the Unseen.

Sex as it is taught and viewed in mainstream patriarchal society is one of the biggest tools for abuse and control. It is often used as a means of perpetuating the power over dynamic and removing an individual's right to autonomy, especially bodily autonomy. One of the foundational principles of Sacred sex is that any sexual act must honor both you and your partner. There is no room for abuse within Sacred sex. It's my belief that if we taught Sacred sex earlier, we could prevent many acts of sexual abuse and assault, among many other benefits. I feel the need to point out that there are some "spiritual" teachers and schools that utilize sex as a form of abuse or as a means to increase their personal power or control. No matter what they call it, these acts are *not* Sacred sex. To clarify, Sacred sex *must* be honoring of all who are involved and be truly consensual.

Even though I know that I can have this experience with any Plant, I have only orgasmed with one other Plant in my waking life. That time was with Stinging Nettle and ki caught me completely off guard. I gently touched Nettle and noticed that ki enjoyed it. Most people are afraid of touching Nettle, but ki simply likes to be treated respectfully. I continued to caress Nettle, loving ki, when I suddenly experienced an orgasm. My focus was on Nettle and not on my body, so I was surprised. My aim is to be of service to the Plants and repair my relationship with Nature. I choose to exchange energy to support the Plant, deepen my connection with ki, and learn from ki. Sometimes the energetic exchange of our connection bubbles up and, rather than direct this toward orgasm or my sexual pleasure, I direct this out to the universe so that our Love and connection can feed the world. In these moments, I am able to feel the Oneness of the universe.

Sometimes when people learn about my experiences orgasming with Plants, they want to learn how to do this, treating these exchanges like a hook-up on a dating app. Engaging with Plants specifically for our sexual pleasure is another form of taking and is out of alignment with Sacred sex. Remember the foundation of Sacred sex is honoring your partner. Again, our culture has an unhealthy relationship with sex. It seems fitting that Plants are willing and able to help us heal our culturalization and awaken our Divine sexuality for they are unabashedly sensual Beings. Remember, those gorgeous flowers are a Plant's reproductive organs. If you spend time observing and learning about Plants, you soon discover that they have many ways of sexual reproduction, which they simply embrace. Plants teach us to let go of shame and judgment and remember that sex literally feeds the world.

Romancing the Plants

Unfortunately, due to trauma including the enormous amount of sexual assault, many people do not know how to engage in a healthy relationship. The Plants, of course, can help us to heal and guide us in learning how to engage with other humans. My dearly beloved Ash taught me how to engage in a process we call Romancing the Plants. Since that time, I have shared this with my students and clients and am amazed at how profoundly they have been affected.

Romancing the Plants is based on a simple concept: you connect with a Plant and treat them as you would a lover. You court them; you touch and caress them gently (asking permission first); you speak sweet words to them; you observe them closely; you give them gifts; you listen to them; you ask what they want and need; in short, you love them and treat them with Love and reverence, just as you do when you first meet a lover. This process came naturally as I was honoring an Ash Tree who radiated Love toward me. I wanted to know how I could honor ki and we began this process. Over time, my Love has only deepened and I discovered that while I was honoring Ash, I was also feeding my Heart and deepening my connection with ki.

When I encouraged my students to Romance the Plants, they were excited—but then some realized that they didn't know how to romance someone. They were never treated this way. Some of them had experienced intense abuse to the point that they no longer felt safe with other humans. I encouraged them through the steps, which included learning how they want to be touched and spoken to and discovering what makes them feel loved. They realized that it was much easier to engage in this way with a Plant who they knew was not going to harm them. Romancing the Plants gave them permission to open their Hearts and experiment. Ultimately, they learned how to recognize the Sacred in another Being as well as in themselves.

As part of this process, I encourage my students to write a poem for their beloved Plant. Poetry is an incredible way to express your Love and create beauty with very few words. Poetry is often taught as an intellectual process, leaving many to feel that they cannot understand poetry, let alone write it. But I promise that you are capable of writing a poem. Through this act of writing a poem for your Plant, you engage in deep appreciation and express this with words. There is no form or rules. You do not need to rhyme or follow a particular pattern. You can ignore punctuation or you can include it in interesting ways. Poetry gives you permission to play with language. It is an amazing way to honor your Beloved.

Below is the poem that I wrote for Ash as we discovered this process of Romancing the Plants. I share this with my students to encourage them to engage in this manner. (Willow understands that I am sharing a poem for Ash in ki's chapter. If I had known how to romance the Plants when I engaged with Willow all those years ago, I am sure that I would have written a steamy and loving poem for ki. Maybe I still will.)

Ash Courting

Oh how I wish
I was a raindrop
Gliding down
Your long, straight body

Moving in and out
Of your crevices
Moistening as I flow
Into your dark places

Taking my time
Willing to have
You burst my bubble
Causing me to become a puddle,
Soaking into you

Or if I may be so lucky
To survive the long journey
Down your glorious Being
Exploring your undulations
Kissing you as I go

May I land at your feet
Soaking into the ground
Flooding the worm holes
Praying that I may be
Sucked by your roots
And find myself in your heartwood

These are both lucky fates
For whichever route,
My boundaries will dissolve
And I will merge into you
Nourishing you and loving you
Through it all

Grief

Life is funny and unexpected. Sometimes something that brings a great deal of pleasure to you can end up causing you so much pain. Romance is an easy example. My experience with Willow was otherworldly and opened me up in a way that I didn't know was possible. Willow played an important part during another time in my life as well, during possibly the most painful experience I have had.

When I was about eighteen months old, my mother was pregnant with my baby brother. Sadly, she lost the baby and due to complications was unfortunately no longer able to have children. However, I desperately wanted a sibling, so, I did the only thing that I knew to do at that time—I prayed. I prayed and I prayed for a sibling.

A couple years later, my prayers were answered and I was given not one, but four siblings, including my brother Michael, who was truly the answer to my prayer. He was only eighteen months older than me. Even though he and our older brother would sometimes beat the shit out of me and absolutely torment me, I loved him like the ocean loves the moon. Until I was in my twenties and had my own family, he was my Sun. I followed him around like a lost puppy.

My brother had a twinkle in his eyes and a laugh like no one else. When he found something funny, he would quickly be rolling on the floor with tears running down his face. It was irresistible, and before you knew it, you would be on the floor laughing with him. This laugh got him out of much trouble and meant that I could never be mad at him for more than a few minutes (and even that was rare).

My sweet, sensitive brother became an addict during his high school years. He was never addicted to anything in particular, though alcohol was a good friend. He mostly enjoyed the escape. His addiction created some incredibly painful and difficult years for him and our family. Somehow, though, he managed to pull himself out of it. He fell in Love. They had a child, who became the Love of his life; I never saw a father like him. He made my Love for and dedication to my children look minuscule.

He was prescribed oxycodone twice within a year for two different surgeries. The first time, I held my breath and prayed, knowing the dangers, but he seemed to have no issue. The second time, however, we weren't so lucky. He recognized quickly that he was addicted to it and asked his doctor for help, but his doctor told him that he wasn't really addicted, he just thought he was. His life spun out of control, and the old addictive behaviors reared up with a vengeance. For the first time in his life, he admitted that he was an addict. He also made an appointment to look into a treatment program. Unfortunately, he died the night before his appointment. He was thirty-six.

The world as I knew it ended on June 8, 2011.

Prior to my brother's death, I didn't understand grief. I believed that people simply transitioned into another life, death was a part of life, and we should celebrate the time we had with people rather than mourn their "loss," for it wasn't a loss at all.

Then grief came knocking on my door. I realized that these were all wonderful thoughts and ideas, but the Heart didn't understand them. The Heart recognizes the absence of a heartbeat. Your fingers long to touch your loved one or to dial a phone and hear their voice.

Suddenly I experienced a crash course in grief. I plummeted into what I call the Abyss of Grief. The world went dark as my Sun disappeared. I did not want to live on this Earth without my brother. I didn't know how I could. Even my Love for my children couldn't keep me here. I spent days on the bathroom floor, my then-husband helping me back into bed because I couldn't walk, only to end up back on the bathroom floor wailing. I wanted to hurl myself into the grave with my brother's casket; my sister's arms tight around me prevented me from doing so. For the first time in my life, I understood alcoholism. I wanted to drink so badly to numb the pain, yet I knew that if I started I wouldn't be able to stop.

At some point, I had to begin to go through the motions of life again. My kids needed to eat. My parents couldn't lose another child. I learned how to take care of others while co-existing in the Abyss. I excelled at driving while hysterically crying.

I have always been a big crier. When we were children, my brothers would make fun of me for it, but I didn't care—I cried. In college, though, I learned that if I was to be taken seriously, I would have to control my tears, so I did. Still, I had several friends who would ask me to watch movies with them because they had a hard time crying and my tears would help them shed theirs. I was a crier and I was comfortable with my tears. However, my crying reached a whole new level after Michael's death. I didn't know what to do with the tears. Fortunately, Nature is always there for us, even when we don't realize it. I started to visit my beloved friend, Willow. Willow kept asking for my tears. She said that she would hold them for me. If I needed more, I would have them. I sat with her and cried, giving her my tears. My tears started to lessen as I began to feel stronger.

While I cried with Willow, I noticed that her branches would wrap around me. I felt held and comforted as if I was in the arms of the Mother. Sometimes her branches would sweep over my head. I felt her soothing me, calming me. I learned that there is a reason why she is called Weeping Willow. I always thought it was because of the shape of her branches. However, Willow helps those who are grieving and weeping. She holds them safely, allowing them to release and transmute their pains. But of course, Willow bark has long been a traditional pain reliever and is what aspirin was originally derived from.

This is a good example of the difference between substances that are derived from a Plant and working with the Plant Spirit. Aspirin can be a good pain reliever, though it is symptomatic, meaning that the aspirin does not change the issue that caused the pain, it simply covers it up. (Yes, it can reduce the inflammation; however, what is causing the inflammation?) Pain is an indicator that something is going on in the body. Usually this something originated in the emotional or spiritual bodies before manifesting in the physical. Since the pain is trying to get your attention, it tends to continue to increase the more you ignore or suppress it. This is why people with chronic pain often discover that their pain medication no longer works and they need to switch to something stronger, which is a dangerous game to play. If we can unearth the original issue that is contributing to the pain, perhaps an abusive childhood or the death of a parent, we can address this issue so that the body no longer needs to respond with pain. This process often is not as easy or quick as popping an aspirin.

Willow Plant Spirit says, "I can hold your pain for you." What Willow knows is that severe trauma and emotional pain are often too difficult for us to carry alone. This is something many of us have a hard time recognizing. We want to keep our pain to ourselves to avoid displaying our weakness or being a burden. When we hold onto and suppress our griefs and wounds, we simply invite them to manifest in our bodies, which they do often as lung issues, heart issues, cancer, fibromyalgia, arthritis, body pain. . . . The truth is that we are communal Beings; we are meant to share the sorrows as well as the joys of life. They are both important experiences that greatly contribute to our well-being.

I have a large, interconnected, motley crew of a family. In the beginning, we all grieved together in a state of shock. However, as time went on, our experiences of grief differed greatly. Part of this is because as a culture, we do not really honor or understand grief. We think it is something that we should process and move through quickly, and where I live, you should be strong as you go through it. However, grief is often a long process, with many mountains and valleys. When we try to take a shortcut, we only lengthen the journey. Combining family dynamics with the different ways of experiencing grief can lead to a potentially volatile situation. I realized that my experience was greatly different from the other members of my family, which is typical of most of my life experiences. Willow gave me the great gift of allowing me to share my grief without adding to anyone else's. Handing my pain to Willow didn't mask the problem, it allowed me to breath and to start to climb out of the Abyss of Grief, which previously felt like an impossibility.

> *Beloved Willow,*
> *Wrap your arms around me*
> *Hide me*
> *Keep me safe*
> *Take my tears from me*
> *There are plenty more*
> *Support me*
> *Heal the pain.*

As I began to ascend from the Abyss, I realized that grief was the price of Love, and ultimately one of its gifts. If I had not felt deep Love, I would not have felt deep grief. I would never trade my time with my brother to reduce the pain. Somehow, this helped to lessen the grief, as it became a lesson in Love. Rather than remaining a victim of grief, I became grateful for the Love of my brother.

This is not to say that if you do not grieve the death of someone you did not Love them. My grandfather died the same year as my brother. I miss him. And I was happy that he passed. He was ninety-nine and had been struggling for the last six years of his life. His death was beautiful and a blessing. It is very different when someone dies suddenly. Of course, our relationship to the deceased also changes the role of grief. My grandparents were married for seventy-three years. For my grandmother, the death of her husband was the loss of her partner, her rock, the person who taught her about Love and defined her life. She grieved her husband's death, even though she was happy he was no longer suffering. My strong, stoic grandmother stood during the viewing and did not shed a tear, believing this would dishonor my grandfather. Months later, on what would have been their seventy-fourth wedding anniversary, my grandmother's grief appeared in the form of shingles, which ended up being the worst case of shingles anyone in our local hospital had ever seen and which nearly killed her.

We must allow ourselves to feel the depth of our grief, to howl and scream and cry a monsoon. This is how we honor our loved ones and how we keep ourselves sane. Ironic, isn't it, that most people are afraid that they will lose their sanity if they allow themselves to express their grief, but it is the repressing of grief that makes us sick and crazy. As Martín Prechtel writes in his beautiful book, *The Smell of Rain on Dust: Grief and Praise*, "Praise and the depth of our grief expressed for one another keeps the world in love. Love is health."[3]

Depression

You do not need to tragically lose a loved one to experience grief. Grief is part of our human experience. I don't know that it is meant to have as large a role as it does. However, one only needs to briefly browse the news to begin to feel grief bubbling up. Entire species are dying. I can witness that the car windshield no longer is covered with insects when I drive at night, like it was when I was a child. I no longer recognize the Landscape of my childhood as it has been paved over and sprouted houses. And then there are the atrocities inflicted on our human kin, especially the children. If we listen, we can hear the cries of our relatives: Salmon, Koala, Elephant, Redwood, Monarch, Amazon Rainforest. They are trying to get our attention. They want us to remember our part in Nature. We can try to ignore the cries, but there is a part of us that continues to hear them. There is a part of us that knows something is missing, that yearns for connection, community, and belonging. We can continue to ignore it, we can continue to grieve, or we can remember. Remember our innate connection with Plants, our innate connection with the wild, our innate connection with air. Remember that we are a part of everything, that we are one, that there is no separation—that we are Nature. This is how we re-member our wholeness.

Until we do this, we are destined to grieve. This grief is often felt as a deep sadness without a name, an emptiness, a hole. It originates from an unidentified source and seems pervasive. We often refer to this as depression. We can medicate with prescriptions, alcohol, food, shopping, or whatever numbs us for a moment. But there is no medication that can erase this for it is caused by amnesia. And you cannot medicate memory into being. Depression is due to a loss of Soul Force energy in one form or another. This is noticeable in the dimness of a person's eyes; their vitality is missing. Sometimes this loss is caused by severe trauma, including generational trauma. However much of depression is a result of our perceived disconnect from Nature, from our very Mother, the Source of all life. For too long, we have been the rebellious and arrogant teenagers who think we know everything and do not need our Mother or other relatives. If we want to live as intact, happy humans, we need to fall on our knees, allow our Hearts to open wide, and pour our tears into the Earth as we ask our Mother for forgiveness. She will grant it; it is already granted. For like any loving Mother, she has maintained the relationship without us noticing.

We may find that as we feel Earth embracing us, more tears emerge. Perhaps it is almost a flood, and we wonder if these tears will ever stop. I encourage you to let them flow. They are cleansing your body. We have been holding them mostly unconsciously. These held tears can manifest as disease inside our bodies. It does not do us any good to keep them, they are not the treasures, the battle scars, nor the weakness that we thought. They allow us to release our walls and the tensions in our bodies as we experience the unconditional Love of our birthright. Our tears are the offerings that bring us back into our beautiful, extended family. As we grieve, we discover that what we have been longing for has been there all along.

There are many Plants who help us to navigate this journey through grief, including St. John's Wort, Elecampane, Cedar, Onion, and, of course, Willow. The Fukushima Daiichi nuclear disaster occurred a few months before my brother's death. A dear friend was connected to a community near there. We sent them Essences for emotional support and protection from the radiation. I made Essences with Plants who volunteered to assist in the healing. Several of them focused on navigating through grief or finding the beauty of life after grief. I had no idea that we were also making these in preparation for my plunge into the Abyss of Grief. All of Nature works as a community. And so, it is no surprise that as Willow helped me to begin my return journey from the Abyss, Rose, who we will meet in the next chapter, joined us.

Exercise: Romancing Your Plant Ally

For this exercise, you want to connect with your Plant as if ki is your lover, your Beloved. You have already experienced many of the components of Romancing the Plants, just not through this perspective.

To prepare for this, you may want to reflect on what makes you feel loved and honored. How do you like to be touched or spoken to? How do you like to be courted? What makes you feel good?

- Move into your Heart space before connecting with your Plant. If you are feeling uncomfortable, breathe with your Plant. Sometimes the most romantic act we can do is to simply sit and breathe with someone. Take your time observing your Plant, noticing and appreciating ki's beauty and form.

- Engage your senses. Perhaps (with permission) take a small bite of an edible portion. Chew slowly, understanding that you are bringing your Plant ally into your body. Their cells are now part of you. Feel the energetic exchange in this. Inhale their scent deeply. Allow this to permeate your cells.

- Speak your Love to your Plant. How do they respond? Imagine your words feeding them, enlivening them. Remember that as you speak, you exhale carbon dioxide which nourishes them. Let your words bathe them in beauty.

◢ Asking permission first, touch your Plant, caressing ki. Let your fingers be an extension of your Love. How does ki want to be touched? Allow your fingers to follow the contours. How lightly can you touch them and still be connected?

◢ As you engage in this way, feel your energy merging with your Plant ally. Feel the Love that you create together. How does your body respond with this exchange? What are you learning about your own needs and desires? How does it feel to be loved as you are?

◢ You can engage like this as often as you like. As you go about your day, take a moment to think of your Plant ally and send them a telepathic note of Love and appreciation.

◢ Write a poem or a Love letter for your Plant ally. Allow your words to pour forth like honey straight from your Heart, honoring and celebrating your Plant lover.

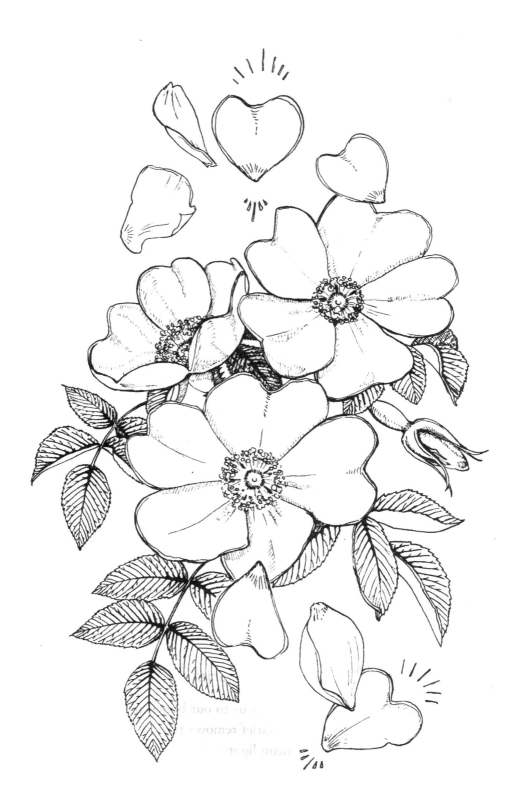

12

❧ Power of Love ❧
Rose

Of all the Plants who helped me through my grief, Rose became my constant supporter. Willow helped me progress to the point at which I was ready for Rose, and when I was, I infused myself with ki in every way possible: Rose tea, Rose glycerite, Rose Flower Essence, Rose water, Rose baths, and time with Rose throughout the day, every day.

Rose became my Heart, helping me to bring my pieces back together. Rose breathed life back into my empty shell. Rose helped me to realign with the vibration of Love. With Rose's guidance, I arose from the Abyss of Grief more awake, alive, and aligned than I was before. My brother's death shook me to my very core. I had been living a life of fear, waiting to be happy. Michael's death taught me that we never know how long we will live, and that we need to make the most out of the time we have, enjoying life and celebrating the abundance of gifts. In so many ways, my brother's death gave me life and I am forever grateful to him, I wish I could hug him and thank him in person.

Embracing Grief

There are gifts in grief. Grief rattles us to our bones, providing us the opportunity to recreate our life. Grief removes the illusions and shows us our priorities, shining like neon lights while we reevaluate our roles and relationships. Grief brings us alive. People often have a great fear of grief. If you are grieving, you may witness people avoiding you or only having peripheral contact. It is as if they fear that grief is a communicable disease. It can be difficult to be witness to someone else's great pain, when there is nothing we can do or say to truly help, and so people try to avoid grief.

If we avoid grief, we avoid life, and we avoid Love. If we do not allow ourselves to grieve fully, there will be a dense curtain between us and the fullness of life. It is the absence of grieving, the absence of processing our grief and traveling through it, that locks us in a state of depression. The real danger here is that we will harden our Hearts and our grief will manifest as physical ailments, while diminishing our Soul expression. If we do not grieve, we pass this burden onto our future generations, poisoning them.

One of the difficult aspects of grief is that there is not a formula or flowchart to follow. Grief is not linear. Everyone grieves in their own way and on their own timeline. Sometimes, too, just when you think you have moved out of grief, you find yourself wailing again. I remember driving to pick up my children one day, feeling happy and thinking, "I have a handle on this grief thing." Just as I thought this, the song that I associate most with my brother started playing. Suddenly I became a ball of tears and realized I was not done grieving.

In order to embrace grief, we need to acknowledge it, name what we are grieving. We need to allow the feeling to move through us without judgment. We may feel sadness or anger or relief or happiness or overwhelm. We may find ourselves screaming or laughing or bawling. We may need to sleep a lot. We may have no appetite or we may want to eat constantly. We may find ourselves inspired to create or we may be paralyzed. We may find that all of our experiences are heightened or everything may be dull and distant. I was unable to read for over a year. I found that I needed to move my body. I would get on my elliptical, put on Pearl Jam's *Ten* (a special album for my brother and me), and exercise while crying hysterically and screaming the songs at the same time.

It's good to cry, wail, and howl. Tears cleanse us. You want to get it out. You may want to have guardians to protect you so that you can focus on releasing. If you are struggling to cry, then go to the ocean or other moving water, or take a warm bath. Water encourages our bodies to release. We may need a little encouragement to get the tears flowing, such as watching a sad movie, or even cutting an Onion.

During active grief, it is important to engage in energy hygiene and receive supportive healing work, such as massage, acupuncture, Flower Essence therapy, or Plant Spirit Healing. If you are able to, grounding will help to bring you back into your body. Spend as much time in Nature as you can; Nature will speak to your Heart. Journaling or creating art may help to express what you are unable to say or even realize consciously. Ceremony is incredibly helpful.

When we are in deep grief, we are the caterpillar who completely dissolves in the cocoon. It may seem as if life is over, but it's only transformation. As you begin to emerge out of the Abyss, it is time to visualize your wings. How do you want your life to be? How do you want to feel every day? What is missing? What do you want to release?

If you can dare to let grief roll you like a stone on the ocean floor, you will emerge with clarity and a glow that is recognizable. Rather than your Heart hardening, your Heart will expand. You will be able to receive, express, and experience more Love than before. If at any time you are needing help, call on Rose. Ki is there to guide you, to support your Heart, and to open your wings wide.

Rose helps to heal the wounds and lightens the load on our Heart. So often, we are afraid of heartbreak. It can be very painful. It is also an opportunity. When we experience heartbreak, we can choose to shut down our Heart, to harden. Rose, of course, would not recommend this, but it is an option. Or we can choose to breathe into the pain and let our Heart expand. As we do, we discover our Heart is not breaking, but growing and stretching. Rose can guide us through so that it is not quite as painful, reminding us to keep our Heart soft and open, for by doing this, we experience less pain overall than if we had hardened our Heart.

The Love of Rose

Tears
Tears
More tears
For what
Why am I crying
Whose tears are these
They are the tears held
The tears unshed
The wounds ignored
The pain stifled
The smiles plastered
They are the pain
The grief
The fears
The unmet needs
They are mine
They are no longer needed
They are the healing
They are the Love of Rose

Power of Love

There is much written and romanticized about Rose, for good reason. Perdita Finn and Clark Strand write, "Roses are very old. Fossils of five-petaled roses have been found in the archaeological record from 35 million years ago—which means they were already there long before hominids evolved."[1] Our love affair with Roses has formed and inspired us for ages; we evolved with them. "If humans planted roses because roses were beautiful, roses taught humans what beauty is. Possibly, roses taught humans what love is."[2] My teacher, Rocío Alarcón, says that Rose was once a master Plant. I think ki still is. In fact, I think Rose is *the* Plant to guide us through our current evolution.

It is widely accepted, even amongst non-Plant people, that Rose is connected to Love. Rose is an incredible support for the Heart. And yes, ki is the embodiment of Love—all forms of Love, not just romantic. Rose helps to awaken that part of us that gnows that Love is the center of everything. And when our Hearts are battered or shut down, Rose holds them in loving compassion so that they can once again open and radiate. Rose reminds us to allow our Hearts to blossom with Love.

Rose carries forth the lesson of Love from Jesus, which is the same lesson of Love that other spiritual teachers have tried to share with us. In essence, this lesson is a reminder that we are the embodiment of Love, that Love is the center of all, and that Love is The Way.

I once found myself in the time of Jesus during a past-life journey. At one point, I was talking with him and could feel his Love radiating to me (and everywhere). He asked me, along with others, to carry forward his message of Love. For days after this journey, I was in a deep depression. I grieved and mourned. During my time in the journey, I could see the possibility of a world filled with Love, and yet it's been two thousand years and his message (and those of his predecessors and successors) has not taken root. Jesus kept telling me to be patient. I didn't understand; how could two thousand years elapse and still we are not treating one another with Love? Then he reminded me that we have increased the level of Love in this world. He had me look back at that life and remember the intense fear. While there is still fear in this world (and sometimes it feels enormously intense), it is not at the level it was back then. This is because people are responding with Love, even if only occasionally or toward those they know. There are some who are consciously working on increasing Love and who radiate this to the world, and that has helped in our communal evolution. Despite the effort it seems to take, we can move into this Love-filled world easily. It only requires a simple shift, almost like flipping a switch.

Rose holds this possibility for us and very gently helps us to open our Heart. We are human and we are learning. It is okay if we respond to situations with anger or act out of fear. Every time we choose to act with Love, we increase the vibration of Love and slowly, inch by inch, we help our evolution along. Michael J. Roads writes:

> . . . the only certainty is Love. The only firm and stable ground is Love. The only place to be is Love. The only springboard is Love. Love—not emotional love—*unconditional* Love. Absolute Love. Divine Love. Love is an earthquake to every probability that could exist. Love shatters all probabilities, creating the certainty of Love. . . . The greater number of people who are Loving and in-their-hearts, the more optimistic the future scenario will be for *everybody*.[3]

Love Defined

We speak of Love frequently and consider ki to be a fundamental part of life. We have numerous definitions for Love, and yet do we really know what Love is? I hold to M. Scott Peck's definition of Love: "The will to extend one's self for the purpose of nurturing one's own or another's spiritual growth."[4]

When we hold this as the definition of Love, suddenly relationships or experiences do not seem so loving—perhaps including those with our own parents. While this may be (temporarily) painful to admit, it is important to look through this lens of Love and reevaluate our experiences. By doing this, we deepen our understanding of Love and healthy relationships, bringing clarity and helping us move forward in a more Love-centered manner. We are no longer confused, thinking that abuse or neglect are part of Love and therefore accepting these in our adult relationships or believing that we deserve these harmful acts. As bell hooks writes, "When we understand love as the will to nurture our own and another's spiritual growth, it becomes clear that we cannot claim to love if we are hurtful and abusive. Love and abuse cannot coexist. Abuse and neglect are, by definition, the opposites of nurturance and care."[5]

This does not mean that our parents and family did not want to love us or didn't try to love us; they were confused and unable to, due to generational and cultural trauma. As parents, we are told that we need to mold our children to be good people and citizens—in other words, to domesticate them. Domestication often requires us to limit, not nurture, our children's spiritual growth (as well as our own). We can recognize the good intentions behind these actions while simultaneously understanding that they were not acts of Love.

I greatly appreciate Peck's definition; it makes our choices and actions clearer. When we hold that Love is about nurturing someone's spiritual growth, the games, the worry, and the blockages disappear. We can stop wasting our time and energy. It is quite freeing. When we commit to loving someone (a romantic partner, a friend, a child, a co-worker), we commit to honoring their spiritual growth, which means that the millions of articles that are written on how to get a partner are pointless. They are not Love. If we want to experience Love, we need to engage in radical honesty. It also becomes easier to accept the ending of a relationship. Of course we do not want to prevent our loved one's Soul growth. If they need to move on to continue their growth, then that is what we want. This is what is best for us as well. It may be painful but not as painful as staying in a loveless relationship. I have supported numerous clients through leaving their relationships. They often feel bad for their former partner or they are made to feel guilty, but the truth is that if one person's Soul growth is stunted in a relationship, both people are harmed. No one benefits from being in a loveless relationship.

Choosing Love

Looking at the definition of Love, "will" implies choice. Our culture likes to romanticize Love by dramatizing stories of falling in Love, meaning that we are helpless or powerless in the face of Love. While Love is a powerful force, engaging in Love requires consciousness. We don't love someone because we have to; we choose to, and we make the choice many times a day. We can just as easily choose to Love a stranger as we can our family or our romantic partners. It is through choosing Love and treating one another with Love that we change the world.

Love is the strongest force there is. Love has an incredible capacity to heal, which is simply bringing us back into wholeness, reminding ourselves of who we are. When we align our lives with Love, our vibration affects others as we walk through the world. We encourage them to remember the truth of who they are. The ripples of Love reverberate out. We can look at the state of the world and be completely overwhelmed or not be able to see a way forward. However, simply by aligning with Love and choosing Love in our actions and interactions, we create a more loving world. If we continue to do this every day, in every interaction, this world will come into form faster than we could imagine.

But let me warn you, this is not the path for the faint of Heart. Choosing Love is challenging. The patriarchy tells us that Love is—or makes us—foolish and weak. In truth, it takes great strength to choose Love, though this is a different type of strength than that modeled by the patriarchy, in which strong means tough, rigid, stoic, fierce, or even aggressive. That form of strength hardens our Hearts and auras and distances us from one another. Rose teaches us how to be soft and strong at the same time. This is the strength that comes from the Heart, the strength of Love. To be soft does not mean to be a doormat. It means that we operate with compassion and empathy, using our Heart intelligence to determine the best way forward for *all*. This form of strength opens us to one another, reducing our burdens and allowing us to be ourselves. Rose's strength is enlivening.

I have long been committed to Love. A few years ago, I asked my guides to show me all the ways in which I was not acting with Love. I was completely overwhelmed by the pain, but Rose encouraged me to continue. It is much easier to respond from a place of hurt or anger or exhaustion than to choose Love in those moments. But I know that if I want to be who I am meant to be and if I want to live in a world that is loving and honoring of all life, then I need to respond from a place of Love in all of my interactions. I still falter, and that's okay—Rose is there to help me choose Love again and again.

Self-Love

Choosing Love is especially important for our interactions with ourselves. So many of us take the limiting beliefs and wounding we've experienced and use them as fodder for our self-critics. Our self-critic has a very real purpose—trying to protect us from being wounded again. However, the internal criticism bathes our cells in hatred and judgment, keeping us from experiencing Love. If we want to create a more loving world, we need to start with ourselves.

When I left my marriage (one of the gifts from Michael's death), I was a broken woman. I had lived with someone with narcissistic tendencies for nearly fifteen years. I was disoriented, and no longer even knew what I enjoyed. I remembered that when I was younger, I felt attractive and confident. For years, though, I thought I was disgusting, an embarrassment, and unlovable. This is what happens when you experience emotional abuse, gaslighting, and other mind games.

I took the adage "no one can love you if you don't love yourself" to Heart. I do not actually think this saying is true; however, I didn't want to risk it on the chance that it was. Consequently, I went into an intense period of learning self-Love, self-acceptance, and self-forgiveness, which included much support and guidance from Rose.

Now I know that if you do not love yourself, you cannot fully love others. This does not mean that we cannot experience Love or that we won't find a partner. But since we are all connected, if you cannot love yourself, you cannot nurture someone's spiritual growth because you are connecting with them through a sense of lack and wounding. When we truly love ourselves, we are able to connect with others from a place of fulfillment.

As I have guided my students and clients on journeys of self-Love, I have noticed that there is a common fear that self-Love leads to narcissism. If you are concerned about this, you needn't be, for it is an impossibility. Narcissism is self-hatred, fear, and trauma hidden under the guise of self-aggrandizement. You cannot love yourself into narcissism.

However, I think that it is possible, with an extensive amount of therapy, to love oneself out of narcissism.

When we love ourselves, we undo the domestication we experienced including the wounds, the limiting beliefs, and the messages that we are not enough. Through loving ourselves, we have the opportunity to experience unconditional Love. Engaging in a practice of self-Love brings healing to our relationships. Through self-Love, we discover Heaven on Earth. We witness that life is miraculously improved. We are suddenly surrounded by amazing people and experience beautiful relationships we wouldn't have imagined before. At least, that has been my experience.

I can hear the critics start when I talk about self-Love. "I do love myself. I'll just love myself more after I lose 15 or 115 pounds" or "I'll love myself once I get rid of this facial hair, or this acne, or this gray hair" or "I'm an addict; I don't deserve to be loved." All of these reasons, all of the self-hate, is manufactured. The truth is that you are Love and worthy of Love as you are at this moment. When the voice of self-hate starts to speak, ask, "Who is profiting from this?" Self-hate and self-criticism are not normal and natural, they are not you. They are byproducts of white supremacy, patriarchy, capitalism, trauma, and a toxic society.

One of the first steps toward self-Love is to recognize the ways the inner critic affects you. I learned this trick from David Dalton to become aware of the criticisms and putdowns we direct our way, both verbally and internally. Every time that you criticize yourself, pinch the back of your hand between the thumb and forefinger, pinching the same spot throughout the day. At the end of the day, evaluate the mark on your hand. This gives a visual representation of the energetic harm we do to ourselves every day. Some of you may cringe at the thought of pinching yourself, yet we rarely stop or redirect the inner critic, who thinks that we deserve these comments.

Self-Love is our natural state. This means that we can overcome negative conditioning and return to our Truth. Self-Love is a journey, not a destination, and as we engage with Love, we discover more about ourselves. Love transforms.

During my deep dive into self-Love, Rose gifted me with a ritual. I have continued to practice this and have shared it with hundreds of students and clients. It is simple and yet transformative.

Exercise: Self-Love Ritual

- Buy a large candle, I prefer a Rose scented candle; however, you can use whatever feels special to you. This candle is only for you.
- Light the candle, ideally every day. As you do, say an intention or prayer, such as, "I light this candle in honor of Love for myself."
- This is your time to experience self-Love. You can sit and meditate with the flame of the candle; as you do, feel yourself surrounded by Love, self-Love. You could do something that feels like Love to you: eat a chocolate, read a book, take a bath, have a nap, engage in self-pleasure, journal, listen to music, create art, stare at yourself in the mirror as you send Love to every part of you. Whatever you do, you want to be aware that you are doing this in Love for yourself. The options are endless; have fun and explore. Give yourself the Love you'd like to receive from a partner, the Love you deserve.
- If you feel stuck or other emotions arise during this, you can always call on Rose to help or perhaps journal about what you are feeling.
- When you are finished, put out the candle. (Some recommend that we do not blow out a magical candle, but snuff out the flame instead.)
- Be sure to thank both Rose and yourself for loving you.

Often our experience with self-Love focuses on our bodies. In our society, there are some bodies that are accepted more than others and some bodies that frankly are more dangerous to have, not because they are any less amazing, but because of the systems of control at the center of our culture. As we begin to love our bodies, our appreciation for other bodies grows: the colors, the shapes, the sizes. What an incredible, beautiful world we live in—our bodies contribute to this.

While we want to love and appreciate every aspect of our bodies, I find it helpful to start with one area. I generally suggest the hands or the eyes. Look at these with innocent perception. Remember all the ways in which they contribute to your life. What joy have they brought? Notice the different shapes, colors, and markings. How incredible they are! Continue to love your hands or eyes until this becomes comfortable, and then expand to another part of your body. Eventually, honor the stretch marks, the scars, and the cellulite. They are beautiful. If you are struggling, then imagine that you are looking at the body of a lover. How would you love this body? Or try starting with pictures of yourself when you were young. Babies and toddlers naturally love their bodies. I remember watching my children delighting in the discoveries of their bodies. It was a very happy day when they could put their toes in their mouth! Sonya Renee Taylor writes:

> You were an infant once, which means there was a time when you thought your body was freaking awesome too. Connecting to that memory may feel as distant as the farthest star. It may not be a memory you can access at all, but just knowing that there was a point in your history when you once loved your body can be a reminder that body shame is a fantastically crappy inheritance. We didn't give it to ourselves, and we are not obligated to keep it. We arrived on this planet as LOVE.[6]

Sometimes when we talk about self-Love, especially in the context of loving our bodies, feelings of judgment and shame creep up because we do not love ourselves or we do not feel good about our bodies. Try as best as you can to meet these feelings without judgment, to hear them, and to know that this is part of undomestication. It takes time to undo the training we've internalized, but I promise you it can be done and that you do not need to change anything about your body. You are beautiful and perfect as you are.

Some suggest that we should focus on accepting rather than loving our body. If that feels better to you, I think it is wonderful. If you can look at your eyes and think they are gorgeous and love them, then that is incredible. Any time that you can truly love and accept any part of yourself, you shift the capitalistic, patriarchal, white supremacist paradigm and that should be celebrated! My wish for you—for this world—is that you truly, completely, deliciously love yourself, for you are Love.

Self-Love includes loving *all* aspects of ourselves, including those aspects that we try to hide or ignore, those parts that we are ashamed of. Some refer to these as our shadow selves. As we engage in self-Love, we see that many of these are coping mechanisms and reactions to our traumas. Some of them are connected to the lessons that we want to learn in this life. Sometimes these aspects are incredible gifts that are simply not valued by the current society. We can go to great lengths to hide these, thinking that they keep us from being lovable. However, they are part of us. Owning them and being honest about them helps others to connect more deeply with us, and allows us to be more authentic. By sharing, we become aware of the gifts of these aspects. Sometimes these parts even become our favorite aspects of ourselves.

If you are struggling with self-Love, go to the Plants. Rose is a great help, but any Plant can guide you through this. Look at the Plant, talk with the Plant. Do they wish that they were someone else? Do they wish that they had a different form? (Well, sometimes cultivated Plants wish for this, but that is again because they have not been allowed to grow true to their nature.) Plants remind us again and again that we are beautiful and that we are Love(d). They continue to remind us of this until we are able to believe it for ourselves. Once we can accept this, we suddenly have more time, energy, and money available to direct toward creating a loving world.

A Message from Rose

You are beauty
You are Love
You are light
You are joy
You are laughter
You are grief
You are transformation

You are you
Beautiful, perfectly imperfect, divine you

Open your heart to me
Let the shackles unbind
Let the fears disappear

As you step into your Being
Embracing all that you are
Following your path

Let my Love hold you
Shine through you
For all to see who you truly are

Slow Down, Come Closer

Rose is well known for ki's gorgeous flowers as well as the thorns. Often, we imbue the thorns with meaning, such as the idea that we can't have pleasure without pain or that Love hurts. But these are simply reflections of our worldview. It's fair to consider the thorns as a form of protection. Rose does help to protect our Heart so that we can keep ki open. However, the message I have received (many times) from Rose's thorns is to slow down and to come closer. Rather than frighten me away, the thorns draw me to Rose and prevent me from running away. I tend to get this message when I'm in a hurry, I'm not paying attention, or I'm trying to avoid something. Rose reminds me that you cannot escape from Love.

Too often we think we have to do everything right now, that speed and time are crucial. We go rushing through life without fully participating or witnessing the wonders. This helps us to avoid our emotions and traumas. If we move fast enough, we don't have to feel anything. Rose reminds us to slow down and feel. (There is the famous adage about smelling the Roses.) As we feel, Rose holds our Heart, allowing our wounds to heal and encouraging us to witness the wonders and joys of life. Rose brings us back into relationship. And ki does so gently and lovingly. I often work with Rose in my healing sessions. It is an incredible gift to witness ki helping humanity and especially my clients. Rose reminds us that we can shift, heal, and evolve with grace. Our experience does not have to be painful and dramatic or traumatic. We can simply unfold like the petals of a Rose bud.

I wonder what would happen if we met others' thorns as a reminder to slow down and come closer?

Healing with Love

Love is the center of my healing practice. However, directly healing with Love is too much for some people to handle. They hold their beliefs of being unworthy or broken, or want nothing to do with Love. It is easier for a person to absorb and accept the healing energies of the Plant Spirits. While all Plants remind us that we are Love(d) and help us to return to this truth, Rose is the ambassador of Love.

We all have traumas, wounds, and limiting beliefs. We say that we want to release these or change these, and yet we tend to hold onto them with all of our might. We identify with them, thinking that they define who we are. Sometimes we even wear these around like a crown or badges we've earned. Rocío Alarcón calls these our most precious jewels because that is how we treat them. These "jewels" refract the light of who we are. They tend to keep us from fully experiencing Love. Rose helps to hold our Heart with Love, allowing us to gently dissolve and release them. Sometimes I call on the energies of Mother Mary or Jesus to continue to support and surround my clients with Love, as many of these "jewels" were given to us as children, and it is comforting to be held in the arms of Mother Mary as we release them. Some of my clients have never felt safe and held in loving arms. Mother Mary reminds us that Love is our birthright. Jesus helps our bodies resonate with Love— unconditional Love. The more aligned we are with Love, the easier it is to choose Love, and the easier it is to heal.

A good portion of my apprenticeship program is focused on expanding my students' capacity for experiencing, absorbing, and transmitting Love. Rose is an important component of this process. We spiral around to meet Rose several times, each time going a little deeper as ki introduces us to the power of Love. At some point in this process, we usually have a Rose blessing ceremony. Each person is blessed by having a Rose slowly and lovingly rubbed over their face and potentially over their body. As this is being done, the giver speaks prayers and blessings of Love that honor the truth and beauty of the receiver. This becomes an ecstatic experience for both the giver and the receiver and even for witnesses. Rose ensures that everyone involved is aligned with Love; there is no avoiding it.

Plant Limpias and Sacred Bathing

Technically, this ceremony with Rose is considered a Plant limpia, though our intention is different from the typical limpia. *Limpia* means sweeping or cleaning. A Plant limpia is a form of energy hygiene where we harvest Plants with prayer to create a bundle, also called a broom. A person's aura and body are swept with this bundle. Generally, the process is accompanied by prayers and blessings. The Plants help to gather unwanted energies and infuse the body with the healing prayers of the Plant Spirits (if they are invited). When the ritual is finished, the Plants are then gifted back to the Earth, ideally far from the house and not in the compost. We do not keep the bundle nor hand it back to the person whose energy was cleared because of the tendency to want to attract these energies back to us. We want the energies to be transmuted. A Plant limpia is wonderful when our energy is feeling out of alignment, especially when we have experienced trauma, shock, or abuse. The Plants help to bring us back into our body.

Sometimes we take a similar bundle of Plants and dip them in water and rather than sweeping the person's aura, we sprinkle them with the water, again saying or singing prayers and blessings the whole time. Water is a good conductor and transmuter. Ki holds the energetic imprint of the Plants and prayers. When the process is complete, we offer the Plants and the water to the Earth to transmute the energies that were cleared. This process is sometimes referred to as Sacred bathing.

Sacred bathing is one of my favorite forms of energy hygiene and is a beautiful way of connecting with a Plant ally. There are numerous varieties of Sacred bathing utilized around the world. The basic components of Sacred bathing are water, Plants, and prayer. The Plants that we pick for a Sacred bath depend on the receiver and the intention. In general, I harvest Plants that do not cause contact dermatitis (avoid Poison Ivy or Poison Oak) and are not too spiky. However, I once experienced a Sacred bath by first getting whacked with Nettles and then having Florida water (a special perfume) spit on me. Sometimes there's a reason to pick a particular Plant. In this case, the Nettles were chosen to help strengthen my energy body.

The impact of a Sacred bath depends on the intention. Generally, the purpose is to clear our auras and our bodies, helping us feel energized and lighter. They can be powerful healing experiences. I often include a Sacred bath when a client has experienced abuse. The process is beautiful and can be extremely empowering. I also include Sacred bathing when my clients have lost their sense of themselves. Sacred bathing helps them to remember and own who they are. Sacred bathing is helpful for almost any situation.

In my classes, we generally do a group Sacred bath. We collect Plants while all saying the same prayer and add them to large bowls of water. Together, we break the Plants into small pieces and remove any sharp or spiky pieces as we sing and speak prayers to the water. I then bless each of the participants by sprinkling the water (and Plants) through their aura, typically giving attention to each of their chakras. You can follow the same process for yourself or with a friend.

Any remaining water from this form of Sacred bathing is kept and, after straining out the Plants, preserved using an equal measure of vodka. I pour this into a spray bottle and give the bottle to whomever the bath was for. They can spray their auras every day, surrounding themselves with the healing and blessings of their Sacred bath.

Another popular form of Sacred bathing is adding the Plants to your bath. Again, you want to harvest them with prayer and intention. You can add them directly to the bath water, which is quite beautiful—and messy. I prefer to put them in a muslin bag. Or you can simmer them in water on the stove for seven to ten minutes, essentially making a strong tea, and pour this into the bath water. Because you soak in this water, you do not want to preserve ki for a spray, although you could reserve some for this purpose before bathing. You can imagine that the blessings and prayers will go out into the world as the water drains.

Pam Montgomery taught me the following prayer that I use for harvesting the Plants. I say this prayer, which originally came from Rosita Arvigo, for each clipping as I harvest. For instance, if I'm harvesting three sprigs of Tulsi, I will say the prayer three times.

> *In the presence of_____ (I say "All that is." You*
> *can fill the blank as you like, for example, "the*
> *Divine," "Love," "God" . . .)*
>
> *I give my thanks to you, _____ (insert the name*
> *of the Plant or, if you do not know, give the Plant a*
> *name such as Beautiful One.)*
>
> *And I trust with all my Heart*
>
> *That you will bring healing to _____ (insert the*
> *name of the person you are collecting the Plants for.)*

You can tailor this prayer or add to it if there is something in particular that you are focusing on.

Whatever form we utilize, experiencing a limpia or Sacred bath with Rose helps us to realign with Love and our wholeness. Rose provides the strength we need to deal with the difficulties of life, while reminding us of the beauty that surrounds us.

Exercise: Sacred Bathing

While Sacred bathing is a wonderful form of energy hygiene, ki is also a great way to connect with your Plant ally.

For this activity, choose which form of Sacred bathing you would like to experience and follow the ritual as described above. This time, you will only harvest your Plant ally. For example, if your Plant ally is Pine, harvest Pine branches to do a limpia or pine needles for a Sacred bath. If your Plant ally is one that you would not like to bathe with (such as Poison Ivy) or you are unable or do not want to harvest them (such as Pink Lady's Slipper), then you can add the Essence of your Plant ally to a bath or spray.

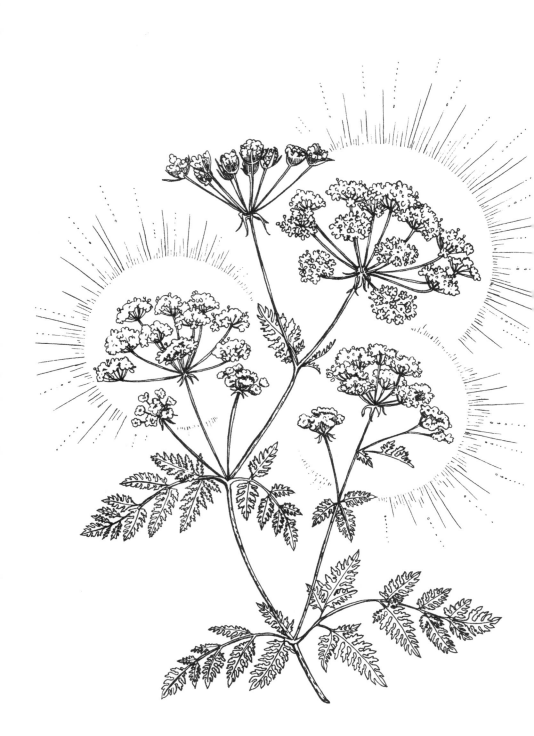

13
⇜ Living to Die ⇝
Poison Hemlock

*P*oison Hemlock may seem like a strange Plant ally to have since ki is deadly. After my divorce, I rented a house in a small town, just blocks from where my paternal grandparents once lived. All of the backyards connected in a row, so that you could stand in my yard and see my neighbors' manicured, perfectly mown yards up and down the block. In the middle of this suburban dream was my small garden. One spring, Poison Hemlock appeared in the center of one of my garden beds. Ki's appearance felt almost obscene. I knew if my neighbors identified this Plant, they would be horrified. Fortunately, they didn't. I couldn't ignore the invitation and thus began my relationship with Poison Hemlock.

Poison Hemlock grows in several areas around Heart Springs Sanctuary, sprouting up in the spring and quickly towering over me. I call ki the Queen, for Poison Hemlock has a royal presence, reminding me to stand in my power. Sometimes we want to make ourselves out to be victims, but Poison Hemlock tells us to own our decisions and stories, accept our power as creators (and destroyers), and to walk with our head held high like the Divine Beings that we are—a perfect ally for going through a divorce.

To the novice, Poison Hemlock's delicate white umbel flowers may seem harmless, but this is the Siren luring you to your death. There are often warnings about misidentifying Poison Hemlock, especially by confusing ki for Queen Anne's Lace (Wild Carrot) or Yarrow. When in doubt, do not harvest or ingest. Personally, I think it is very easy to notice the differences between these. Where I live, Poison Hemlock dies down by mid-Summer and Queen Anne's Lace blooms in August. One of the biggest identifiers for Poison Hemlock is ki's purple spotted stem (sometimes it's described as red). This coloring on a stem is often a signature for a poisonous Plant.

Overcoming Fear

As I wrote in an earlier chapter, when my brother died, I realized that I had been living a life of fear. Fear dominated me from a young age. I know that a good portion of the fear was part of my domestication and inherited from my family, Ancestors, and culture. Still, I allowed fear to keep me from living the life I truly wanted to live. Now that I had recognized that life is exceedingly short, I wanted to experience as much as I could. Fortunately, at a conference that summer (where I also met Pam Montgomery), I participated in a class with ALisa Starkweather. I do not remember what the class was about, but I do remember ALisa talking about fear and, particularly, the pervasive fear of being burned at the stake. They shared that, at some point, they had stopped caring. ALisa said, "So what?! Are you going to kill me? Go ahead. You can't kill my Soul." Those powerful words continue to guide my life. If I'm no longer afraid of death and torture, what can stop me from living the life I want?

There are many other fears, and they do continue to pop up. But if we can eliminate the fear of dying as well as the fear of not being loved, we greatly reduce the amount of overall fear in our lives. If we want to live a life of Love, we need to choose Love over fear again and again. There is power in fear. Fear diminishes us, allows us to be controlled, and contributes to separation and othering. Fear causes contraction while Love creates expansion.

What I am referring to as fear are the worries that have no basis in reality. A common acronym is False Evidence Appearing Real. There are times when fear is appropriate, but I tend to think of it in these instances as discernment more than actual fear. Discernment tells us we should not go on this trip. Later we discover that there was an accident, or we got sick, or there was a family emergency. Fear could also tell us not to go on a trip, but the vibration, the energy of the feeling is completely different. With discernment you simply know something isn't right or feels off. With fear, there is a contraction and, if you can be honest with yourself, you will often notice that something is triggering it. It may take time to recognize the difference, but I assure you it is worth it. Of course, Plants can assist us in this. We can also ask ourselves if a particular reaction is in alignment with Love. Love knows no fear.

This may seem like a contradiction, for we have all experienced fear around Love, but that is a reaction from our conditioning and our wounds. Love encourages us to be brave. If we want to truly live a life aligned with Love, we need to walk through the flames. One of the best ways for dealing with fear is to identify it. Give fear a seat at the table. So often we try to ignore fear, which only makes it louder. Look at the fear, name the fear, thank the fear, and continue on; most likely you will find that the fear no longer has a power over you.

Sometimes we make "good" choices because of our fear. However, if they are fear based then they are not in alignment with life and Love. For instance, we may choose to eat organically because we are afraid of the effects of the pesticides. This means that as we eat our food, we are feeding ourselves fear. We can also choose to eat organically because we see this as a way of loving our bodies while honoring Plants, the farmers, and Earth. The same action with different intentions has different effects. There is much in the environmental movement that is fear based. Ultimately, these actions will not help us to create a better world. Instead, we need to respond with Love. We honor Earth, water, and Plants because we love them and want to live in right relationship with them, not out of fear for our future.

Fear of Dying

Our culture is obsessed with dying. By obsessed, I mean consumed by fear. Yet death is a natural part of life. We work so hard at avoiding death that we sometimes need to ponder, are we actually living life?

Our obsession with death extends to the bizarre act of burials, which involves filling a body with preservatives before burying it in a sealed coffin designed to keep the body from decomposing. Decomposition is a part of the life cycle. Ironically, by preventing ourselves from becoming compost we prevent our bodies from continuing with life. Our bodies are made of many different organisms—we are a universe of one. Many of these organisms continue to live after we are considered to be dead, which is why we use preservatives. In a natural death environment, our bodies would continue to feed life, perhaps through a fungus or mold or earthworm or scavenger. Our body becomes part of their body just like the food that we eat becomes part of us. Thus, the circle of life continues.

Everyone else in Nature allows their body to feed others. Only humans do not want to be considered as worm food. Our burial rituals continue the myth of separation. Fortunately, more areas are beginning to allow natural burials or composting pods. Offering our bodies to Earth is literally a way to feed our relations. It is an offering of Love.

We not only fear our own death, we also fear the death of those around us. Sometimes these fears are paralyzing or keep us from connecting deeply with others. As always, when there is a need, a Plant appears. Poison Hemlock helps us to overcome our fear of death. Poison Hemlock reminds us that death is inevitable and not the ending that we fear. Death is a transformation of form. Our Souls live on.

Poison Hemlock helps us move beyond our fear of death to fully embrace the gift of life. This can be helpful at any stage in our journey but especially if our fear is paralyzing us or if our time of death is close and we are afraid to face it. I have been blessed to witness the crossing over of friends, clients, and family members. It is a Sacred and sometimes challenging time. What I have noticed is that those who are afraid of death tend to struggle the most during this transition time. Sometimes their fear is due to strong beliefs about the afterlife. Sometimes they see death as a failure. Sometimes they are concerned about what will happen to their family, business, or even money. Whatever the reason, when we resist, we create difficulty. Poison Hemlock helps us to let go, accept, and embrace death.

Now, I want to be absolutely clear that when I am talking about Poison Hemlock helping us, I am referring to ki's Plant Spirit and Flower Essence. Poison Hemlock is poisonous in even minute amounts (ki killed Socrates). I once was teaching a group how to assist people transitioning from this world. I shared the information about Poison Hemlock helping to overcome fear of death. One of the participants asked how I used this: as a tincture, a tea, an Essence? I laughed and said, "If you give them the tincture, be sure that you do not leave any fingerprints or identifying marks." They just looked at me. I responded, "You would kill them. And that is one way of quickly overcoming their fear of death. But perhaps it would be better to work with the Plant Spirit or Essence."

Death as Failure

Sometimes we consider death to be a failure. This is bizarre since death is inevitable. We will all die at some point. If we hold this belief, then we are all destined to fail. A related belief is that the goal is to live as long as we can. I would argue that our goal should be to live as well and as fully as we can.

Death is not punishment. Nor is death a failure. Often this belief is connected to a person dying from a disease. They think that if they were good enough or prayed enough or tried enough healing techniques they would not die from their disease. Their family members may think that if they had followed this diet or taken this supplement, they wouldn't have died. To me the question is, did they learn what they needed to learn?

Every disease has a gift. We often miss them because of the belief that illness and disease are solely bad. Illness can offer opportunities, however. Lyme disease was an opportunity for me to make myself a priority. Cancer can be an opportunity to reprioritize one's life or reestablish healthy boundaries. Heart disease can provide an opportunity for getting in touch with and expressing one's emotions. These are generalizations; the particular lessons of a disease are dependent on the person. Michael J. Roads writes, "So often illness becomes a pivotal point in a person's spiritual growth; pain and sickness can awaken a person's deeper sensitivity to the world around them. Pain and sickness is often the only way a person will slow down long enough to listen to their inner voice."[1]

Illness is considered bad because it is a disruption. It interferes with work, family, school. It interferes with our productivity—the biggest sin in capitalism. In my world, however, illness is a message from the body. My role is to help my clients to interpret the message. Sometimes we experience illness because we are out of alignment with our Soul. There may be a lesson to learn. Sometimes illness is a preparation for our evolution; I learned when my children were young that they would have a fever right before moving into their next stage of development and I've noticed that I often emerge from a fever with renewed clarity and awareness. Illness may be our body's way of saying we've been doing too much and need to rest. Sometimes illness is the result of malevolent magic or poor energy hygiene. Our body may be trying to draw our attention to a disturbance in our emotional or spiritual body, such as a trauma that needs to be healed or a blocked emotion. Illness can be a result of unhealthy relationship dynamics. Sometimes it provides an excuse for avoiding our traumas or engagement with life. Our illness may occur because the Earth is being poisoned. Looking at illness as a message rather than something that is wrong with us changes our reaction. Ideally, we get curious and listen to what our body wants us to know. Of course, sometimes we just don't know.

I have witnessed people distort this idea into an attack on someone who is ill, essentially accusing them of consciously choosing to be sick, or suggesting that they should simply will themselves well again. No one needs to be shamed for their illness. While illness may bring us lessons and go beyond the physical ailment, in general people do not consciously choose to be sick; in the rare cases when they do, then they need support and Love, not shame. I remember emerging from a week-long fever to be accosted by someone who said, "Why do you want to be sick?" Fortunately, I knew not to take this personally and that they had good intentions even if they were confused.

Looking at illness as a message invites curiosity. It provides an opportunity for healing on a deeper level than the mere reduction or resolution of symptoms. Even if we understand and address the root issue, the illness or the dis-ease may persist. There is a difference between healing and a cure. Healing does not mean the absence of death. Sometimes a disease is required for our healing and sometimes death is part of our healing process. We need to change our perception that life is something we can win or lose at; this is part of the outdated belief of survival of the fittest. There is nothing to win or lose. Life is not a competition. Life simply is. Before coming into this life, we agreed to learn certain lessons to assist our evolution. If we do not learn them in this lifetime, we will have another chance. There's no judge or scorekeeper.

Fear of Aging

Our obsession with avoiding death can be seen in the large number of anti-aging products on the market. We do not want to look "old." We want to be young and full of life. We fight getting older by coloring our hair, lying about our age, and pushing our bodies too far. When we talk about getting older, we usually lament and focus on what we are losing: our hair, our waistlines, our memory, our eyesight, our energy, our sexual drive, our bladder function. My Mimi frequently tells me, "Getting old is not for the faint of Heart."

Thinking that we need to stay young and trying to overcome our age contributes to the separation myth, ignoring the natural progression of our body. Even more, it prevents us from embracing the gift of aging. There are gifts for every phase of life.

Our society does not value the gifts of old age because we value productivity and productivity tends to decrease as we get older. But there is so much more to life than productivity. Throughout my life, my Mimi has always been wise, sharp, funny, and loving. Now, though, there is a softness and sweetness that wasn't there when I was younger. She exudes Love and her eyes have a light to them that wasn't there before. She is still sharp and witty and more playful than I remember her being when I was a child. She is also bedridden and therefore, by cultural standards, not productive. One could even argue that she's a drain on society. Yet if our work in this world is to increase the amount of Love, then my grandmother is one of the most productive. She brightens the life of anyone who comes in contact with her. Her age frees her of the burdens and expectations that we tend to think are important in life but which keep us from expressing Love. She no longer has the illusion that life is long and time plentiful. Therefore each moment is to be enjoyed as much as possible.

Indigenous cultures regard their Elders with a high level of respect. As we transition through the phases of life, we ideally gain wisdom and perspective, becoming Elders who share our journeys' lessons with others. When we come into this world, we continue our strong connection with the spiritual world, and slowly transition to full incarnation on Earth. As we get older, the reverse occurs and our channels of communication with the Spirit world become stronger. We become the visionaries and the sages. At least, we have the potential of experiencing this. Everyone who lives long enough will transition into old age, but not everyone will become an Elder. An Elder is someone who has done (and possibly continues to do) their personal work, aligns with Nature, and chooses Love. They have navigated the turmoil of life and emerged softer, clearer, and with a bigger Heart. Becoming an Elder is an honor not everyone experiences.

Buyer's Remorse

Another way our obsession with death manifests is through suicide ideation and the idea of wanting to go "Home." These are quite common and I refer to them as "buyer's remorse." When we are in the spiritual world considering life, we make agreements about the lessons that we want to learn with this lifetime. In this place, we know who we are, we recognize the Love and support around us, and anything seems possible. For most of us, being born initiates an amnesiac response. For some, this occurs immediately; for others, it happens slowly, over a longer time. We begin to forget who we are. We forget that we are surrounded by Love and support. We forget the lessons that we signed up to learn. We even forget that we wanted this experience and waited a long time to be born.

As we grow and become older, the amnesia tends to strengthen. Often our lives are full of and guided by other amnesiacs. Our lessons, which seemed so simple in the other world, now feel like torture. We want out. We even say, "I didn't sign up for this!" We may begin to experience suicidal ideation such as fantasizing about calamities or ways of ending our life, or fall into a deep depression of Homesickness.

While buyer's remorse is common, it often goes undiscussed by people who are experiencing it, partially out of fear of being hospitalized. This fear and therapists who hospitalize their clients at any mention of suicidal ideation prevent us from sharing our authenticity and from healing. Buyer's remorse energetically appears as a person who is only partially in this world, as though they are standing on a threshold with part of their body in this world and part in the other world. This prevents them from fully experiencing life. It also makes it difficult for them to heal—on all levels. When I see this in my clients, I encourage them to consider making a commitment to this life and learning their lessons.

Suicidal ideation is often a coping mechanism, helping us to feel that we have some control over our lives. It can signal that we are experiencing a flashback to a prior trauma. Pete Walker writes, "Passive suicidality is typically a flashback to early childhood when our abandonment was so profound, that it was natural for us to wish that God or somebody or something would just put an end to it all."[2] We can view these feelings as an invitation to focus on healing our trauma. If you do not trust sharing your feelings of suicidal ideation with your therapist, please find another therapist. A good therapist helps you feel comfortable and safe to share any thoughts and feelings.

There is a large difference between passive suicidal ideation and active suicidality. If you or someone you love is preparing to actively attempt suicide, then please seek immediate assistance. Free, confidential help can be found by calling the national suicide hotline at 988 or visiting 988lifeline.org online.

I have often found that the most sensitive Souls can be prone to suicidal ideation or Homesickness. I have had these feelings, and they were generally provoked by the overwhelm of what I saw as a world filled with hardness and hatred. In the midst of a somewhat near-death experience, I made a conscious choice to stay in this world. I now know that this is where I am meant to be and where I want to be. I still become saddened by the hate and violence and I still miss my "Home" sometimes, but I recognize these feelings as signs of depletion. I then spend time with Plants and my Guides to feed my Heart and Soul.

When we experience this buyer's remorse, our lens is focused on the pain in the world. The Plants, including Poison Hemlock, help us to refocus, to see the beauty. They help us to re-member who we are. They remind us that we did sign up for this. Once we recognize the lessons that we wanted to learn, they no longer seem so difficult. We are blessed to be alive at this incredibly special time for humanity on Earth. We have more Love and support available to us than we can even imagine.

Shamanic Journeying

Poison Hemlock entices us to explore the Underworld. For many people, the only world, the only reality is the one that we can see with our eyes and explore with our bodies. And yet, there is so much more than this reality. We refer to these other worlds as the Unseen. The Unseen is vast and limitless. We can explore and experience this during our dream state, though most of us do not have conscious control over our dreams. However, we can consciously connect with the Unseen by engaging in a shamanic journey.

A shamanic journey allows us to move outside of time and space and to experience the Unseen. When we visit the Unseen, we may experience a different perspective, gain wisdom, or receive healing. There are many types of shamanic journeys. Often, an instrument or sound is used to help shift our brainwaves from beta (ordinary consciousness) to theta (the dream state). Theta brain state is creative, connected to our subconscious, and open to the wisdom of the universe. When we are in this state, we simply gnow.

The word *Shaman* specifically refers to spiritual healers from Siberia. It originates from the Manchu-Tungus word *šaman,* which means "one who knows."[3] However, the term has been used to refer to spiritual healers around the world. Unfortunately, shamanism has been co-opted by the mainstream and one can now take a weekend or online course and call themselves a Shaman. For me, being a Shaman is a life-long endeavor that requires great responsibility and dedication. I have been blessed to have encountered a number of Shamans, though they would mostly refer to themselves as Curanderos. While I have dedicated my life to my spiritual and healing practice and to guiding others on their journeys, I do not feel that my training nor dedication is at the same level of these amazing healers, many of whom were chosen when they were toddlers to carry forward the family tradition. Therefore I do not refer to myself as a Shaman, nor is this someone I aspire to be. My aspiration is to follow my own spiritual path and be me.

Having said that, I believe that each of us has an innate connection to the Unseen and that it is in our best interest to cultivate this relationship. When we do, we have a greater understanding of the world and our place in ki. Cultural appropriation is real and if we want to heal, we need to recognize the forms it can take. There are also foundational truths and sometimes tools that were understood and utilized in cultures around the world, such as using sound to alter our state of consciousness. In my classes, I generally refer to this as "journeying," for that is what we do—we go on a journey from our normal state of consciousness to somewhere else. (In the context of this book, we are journeying to meet with the Spirit of our Plant allies.) But simply saying "journeying," as in traveling somewhere, can be confusing; therefore, I sometimes refer to this practice as shamanic journeying because it is a recognized term. Perhaps we should call this practice sound journeying.

The exercise at the end of the chapter helps you journey to meet your Plant ally. What follows here is a more in-depth discussion of the journeying process, which you can refer to as you prepare for this practice.

We always set Sacred space before journeying. This creates a container that allows us to let go and explore. You may want to ask a Guide or helpers to join you. Your Wise One is always there, even if you do not know them. Some people are convinced that they cannot do this or, more precisely, they are not good enough or spiritual enough to have a journey, but you are and you can. One piece of advice is to use your imagination.

Remember, we create our life with our imagination. If you are having difficulty becoming immersed in the journey, simply allow yourself to imagine, "If I were to go on a journey, what would it look like?" Usually, once you engage with your imagination, everything begins to flow. It is important to know that you are always in control of your experience. If there is something that you are not comfortable with, you can leave or change the scenery, though you may want to be curious about the discomfort.

This is a time of engaging with innocent perception. You want to begin your journey with no expectations, including expectations of how you will experience the journey. There are different ways of experiencing them and they are all valid and wonderful. Some hear their experience while others feel it in their body; for others it is like being in a dream, and some have incredibly vivid images, like they are watching a film. When we journey in groups, there is a tendency of valuing the filmic experience as better than the others, which is not accurate. It does not matter what form your journey takes—what matters is the information that you receive (which is held in our body and sometimes takes years to fully understand). How you experience journeying may change as well. When I first learned to journey, I heard everything, but then my experience became kinesthetic and I felt it in my body, and later still I started seeing my experience. Now I tend to experience a combination, but I have learned to simply accept the form.

If you are having difficulty, acknowledge it without judgment or applying meaning to the difficulty (such as "I can't do this" or "I'm not good at journeying"). I have experienced thousands of journeys and I still have times when it just doesn't work. Usually this occurs when I am overwhelmed or my mind is focused on something else. The idea is to allow the drum or sound to soothe your brain, relax your body, and open you to the Unseen world. But our brains are powerful and sometimes we do not allow ourselves to relax. It can be helpful to ground or stretch before your journey, maybe even do a breathing exercise to help calm your brain. You want to create a comfortable nest. I like to lie on a yoga mat, covered by a blanket with a pillow under my head Sometimes I use a bolster under my knees. Some prefer an eye mask to block out any light.

Sometimes we may fall asleep during a journey. Journeying in the morning and when we are rested helps to avoid this. Journeying after a large meal makes us more likely to fall asleep. If you feel that you might fall asleep, try sitting or even standing or walking during your journey. If you come out of the journey before it is complete, simply listen to the drum or instrument and allow the sound to take you back.

If you are prone to dissociating from your body, then some caution is needed. You may find that you really enjoy the experiences of shamanic journeying, and it can become another form of dissociation itself. Be mindful if you are feeling pulled to spend more and more time within the Unseen worlds. You may also want to have someone there to witness you as you journey, at least until you are a proficient journeyer. They could even drum or guide you. Mostly you want them there in case you do not want to come back when the journey is over. This is a rare occurrence, although I have witnessed it. If you are guiding someone and they don't want to come back, touch their feet and gently call their name. If they still do not come back, rub their arms, back, and, if necessary, legs while you continue to say their name and tell them that it is time to come back into their body. Once they do, stay with them. They may be scared or incredibly sad at leaving the other world.

As I said, the Unseen is vast and limitless; therefore, having questions or a destination in mind helps to direct the experience. Just as in our dreams, symbolism is an important feature of our journeys. Again, it can sometimes take years to understand a particular aspect. Writing down our journeys helps us remember and understand them. Have your journal next to you so that when the journey ends you can easily reach it and start writing. Just like waking from our dreams, we want to be quiet and move as little as possible, which helps us to retain the information and energy of our theta state. Fast movements and loud noise will quickly move us back into beta brainwaves, making it easier to forget our experience. We still had the experience and it is there, but may not be available for our conscious mind.

A common question is, "What if I'm making this all up?" My response is to simply experience your journeys. Over time, you can evaluate if the information or healings that you received were helpful. As with anything, the more you journey, the more comfortable you will be journeying. I still have moments when I doubt the information that I receive, usually when it is related to my clients. When I share the information with them, however, they are surprised and confirm what I have shared.

Shamanic journeying is one of my favorite tools for connecting with the Unseen and getting a different perspective or receiving guidance. This technique has been an enormous benefit in my life. I have not always wanted to hear the information that my Guides shared with me, but they were accurate and, in the end, I've always been grateful.

One last bit of advice: this is a journey. However you go to your destination, you want to return the same way to come back to your body and then into the room where you started. I invite my students to tap the sides of their body and say their name to themselves three times. This helps them to return fully. Oh, and have fun!

Greenbreath Journey

Breathing gives us life, but we frequently ignore the breath's capability for changing consciousness. *Spiritus* is the Latin word for breathing. Our breath is intimately connected with Spirit. We can combine different breathing techniques to enhance a shamanic journey for specific purposes. One of my favorites is a process called the Greenbreath Journey, created by Pam Montgomery.

A Greenbreath Journey is a seventy-two minute guided journey set to music that utilizes activated breathing. The breath that we use helps to create a high frequency that shatters stagnant energy, old patterns, illusions, and stuck emotions. Through this process we can experience spontaneous healing, other dimensions, and an intimate connection with our Plant ally. Ultimately, a Greenbreath Journey helps us to remember who we truly are.

Experiences with a Greenbreath Journey can be intense, healing, blissful, peaceful, and ecstatic. Some people wail and howl, some dance, some lie still, some laugh, some cough up old stuff, some do all of these.

Pam's ecstatic experience with White Pine, that I mentioned earlier, occurred through a Greenbreath Journey.

Through the process of a Greenbreath Journey, we move into the deep, intimate relationship with our Plant ally to the point that there is no separation between us. We become the Plant and the Plant becomes us.

Several of the messages and experiences that I have shared in this book came to me via Greenbreath Journeys. I love when I can experience a Plant via a Greenbreath Journey. That being said, this is a very special journey and one that I do not do often.

As much as I love experiencing a Greenbreath Journey, I also love guiding people through this process. It is a blessing to witness someone releasing and healing what no longer serves them and embracing their truth. If you ever have the chance of experiencing a Greenbreath Journey, I highly recommend them.

A Greenbreath Journey is usually one of the culminating activities of a Plant communication weekend. While this is not something that I can share in this book, it is an incredible tool for gaining insight into your Plant ally's gifts and strengthening your relationship with your Plant ally (as well as yourself). Maybe one day you will be able to experience a Greenbreath Journey and then you will understand why I love them so much. No words can explain the incredible gift that Pam Montgomery has given us by bringing forward this technique.

Our Greatest Fear

Poison Hemlock is a guide into the Underworld and the cosmic realms. My experience sitting with ki was extremely deep, powerful, and otherworldly. It wasn't until I was writing this book that I realized I never journeyed with ki, which is an anomaly for me. Journeying with Plant Spirits is one of my main forms of communication. I, of course, rectified this. My journey with Poison Hemlock was similar to my earlier experiences, though ki highlighted a gift that I had forgotten.

As we met in the Underworld, I saw Poison Hemlock's regal self, standing in ki's power and beauty. Poison Hemlock said, "People try to demonize or misunderstand me, but that's on them. I know my truth and gifts and am unfazed by these depictions. I will not bow to their fear." Then Poison Hemlock showed me ki's connection with Hekate. Hekate is a Moon Goddess associated with the Underworld, crossroads, and crone-ship, among other attributes. Many fear Hekate for her fierceness. My experience is that she is quite loving. Yes, there is a "tough Love" aspect; Hekate will not suffer fools and she sees right through our smoke and mirrors. Hekate understands what we are capable of and won't let us settle for less. Poison Hemlock pointed out that Hekate is also demonized and feared because she knows who she is and embraces her gifts and power.

Poison Hemlock then showed me how the same is true for truly powerful people, especially women. Ki shared, "You need to stand in your Truth and go about your life without paying them attention." Poison Hemlock reminded me of Marianne Williamson's famous quote: "Our deepest fear is not that we are inadequate. Our deepest fear is that we are powerful beyond measure." Sometimes we try to make ourselves small to fit in or maintain situations or relationships. We are afraid to be seen or to shine too brightly. Or we make ourselves small because of limiting beliefs. We do not think that we are worthy of more or we don't want to take up too much space. We limit our dreams or settle for less.

No one benefits from our smallness. We are living at a time of great change. Poison Hemlock encourages us to stand in our truth, embrace our gifts, and shine. The Earth needs us to own our power; this is not about ego or grandiosity. We are being asked to stretch ourselves, dream big, dream with others, and imagine a new way of living in alignment with Nature.

Poison Hemlock helps us to find and embrace our special role. Again, we can get caught up in a hierarchy, thinking that our gifts either aren't valuable or perhaps are more important than others. We each have a place in the Whole; we are each important. Whatever your gifts are, utilize them, share them, stand in the truth of your Being, and shine. The more you stand in your radiant power, the more you encour-age others, and the more you attract the people and opportunities who are most in alignment with your Soul.

Exercise: *Shamanic Journeying with Your Plant Ally*

This is an opportunity to meet the Spirit of your Plant ally and ask them questions or perhaps receive healing or a gift. It is best to do this journey in the morning when you are less likely to fall asleep. Use the following link to download the audio track that accompanies this exercise:

audio.innertraditions.com/cowipl

- To prepare, smudge or clear your space and aura, setting Sacred space. Ground yourself, and then access your Heart space.
- Create a nest for yourself. You might lie on a mat or other soft surface, with pillows and blankets. Do what feels comfortable for you.
- With the recording, I will guide you down to the Underworld. You will meet your Wise One there and ask them to visit the place where the Spirit of your Plant ally lives. Generally, Plant Spirits live in the Underworld, but it is possible that they will take you somewhere else.
- At this point, I will drum for you. Allow yourself to simply experience. If you are stuck, then call on your imagination. Where would your Plant Spirit live? What would your Plant Spirit look or sound like? Engage your senses.
- While you are with your Plant ally, ask them questions, sense their energy, or simply spend time with them. It is possible that they may offer you a healing or a gift. If you need help, you can ask your Wise One or Plant ally (or other guides and guardians) for assistance at any time.
- When the drumbeat changes, that is your cue that it is time to return. I will guide you back to your Wise One and then back to where we started.
- When you return, draw or write about your experience in your journal. Remember to try to be quiet and make as little movement as possible to help you retain your experience.
- A note about your Wise One: they will be there even if you have never consciously met them before. If you prefer, you could do a journey to meet them before the journey to visit your Plant ally.
- If you are an experienced journeyer, feel free to listen to your preferred music or follow your own way to meet the Spirit of your Plant ally.

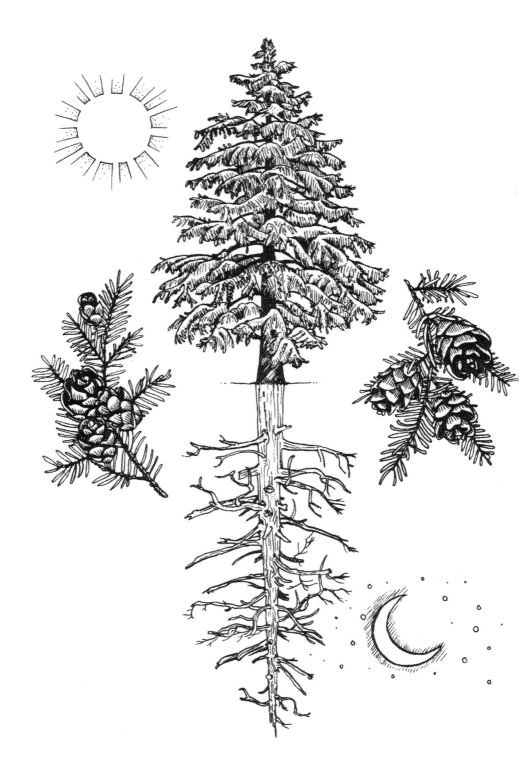

14

ꙮ Everything Changes ꙮ
Eastern Hemlock

*A*gain, Plants come into our lives in many different ways. My relationship with Eastern Hemlock began with ki's wood. When we were building our strawbale home, Hemlock wood was recommended for the skirting around our crawl space. We loved this wood so much that we got more for the attic floor/bedroom ceiling, doors, and other accents. Days spent measuring, cutting, and installing Hemlock captured my Heart; I wanted to know this Tree. While Eastern Hemlock is native to where I live, ki was fairly elusive. Many years later, I wanted to show my gratitude and desire to be in deeper relationship by planting a circle of Eastern Hemlock as the beginning of a Sacred grove. Sadly, most of the Trees did not survive the first year and I left the farm shortly afterward.

I was excited when I discovered Hemlock Trees at Heart Springs Sanctuary. I finally had access to the physical Tree. The Hemlock Trees who grow here intrigue me. They have a tendency to hide in plain sight. I know exactly where they grow, and yet sometimes I cannot see them nor find them. We do not live in a Forest or dense thicket, yet these Trees are mysterious. They are not flashy nor do they grab my attention. They continue to guide and teach us and remain incredibly patient as we blunder along our way.

A couple of years ago, my Love introduced me to what has become one of my favorite places, an old growth Forest a few hours from here where large Hemlock Trees, some of whom were alive before the colonists arrived, grow. There is something magical that occurs when you enter a Forest of old Trees. I feel this whenever I visit the Redwoods in California and I felt it in this Forest. Time shifts, things become clearer, my body relaxes, my Heart opens, and I can feel myself moving into the dreamtime. I begin to sense the possibilities of this world, what life could be like if we re-membered our part in Nature. The domestication and human conditioning including the generational traumas and limiting beliefs melt away, and I sense who I am. I am given a pause. Mostly, I feel deep, unconditional Love.

Sometimes we can know a person for years or even decades and yet we don't really know them. They are a part of our life, but our knowledge of them is superficial. Then sometimes we have an experience that allows them to reveal themselves to us or perhaps we finally see them for who they are. This was my experience with Hemlock. Once I met Hemlock in ki's native habitat, we were able to truly connect. Something shifted within me. I can still sense the Forest and some of the individual Trees with whom I spent time. Sometimes when I need guidance or inspiration or just to remember, I spend time sensing the Hemlock Forest. Ki lives within me.

As I said earlier, the beauty of working with Plant Spirits is that we can work with these Beings anywhere, at any time. We are blessed to be able to have numerous Plants growing near us, some far from their native habitat or climate. As I write, I have Aloe and San Pedro growing in front of me and a large African Milk Cactus growing next to me. I have met Aloe and San Pedro in their natural habitat. While I am grateful to have these Plants here with me, I know that they are not even close to their potential. Plants in their native environment, who have grown without human interference, offer incredible insight. They are quite different from cultivated Plants. There is a context for Plants in their native environment; they are surrounded by the Beings who have helped to form them. When we meet them, we understand their fullness and their potential. It is a moment of awe. It is similar to visiting the Land(s) of our Ancestors; suddenly we have a deeper understanding of our family and ourselves. We are shaped by the Land and the other Beings with whom we share that Land. These places have helped to form our DNA, and the same is true for Plants.

Despite sharing a common name, Eastern Hemlock (*Tsuga canadensis*) is a very different Plant from Poison Hemlock (*Conium maculatum*). Eastern Hemlock is a slow growing conifer who also prefers growing near water. Eastern Hemlocks are pioneers; they were among the first Trees to move north after the glaciers melted. Now these ancient Ancestors are dying due to infestation of the Hemlock Wooly Adelgid, a tiny aphid-like insect.

Quieting the Interference

Before entering the Forest, I ask permission. We humans seem to think that we should be able to go wherever we want, especially if there is a path. It is another way of enacting dominion over Nature. In our fast-paced world it is not feasible to ask permission before entering different Lands; our cars pass through before we can utter the words. However, when I move at a human pace, I recognize that I am a visitor and knock on the metaphorical door. I do this by simply quieting myself and asking internally if I may enter. If I receive a yes, I enter. If not, I stay out. We need to respect the wishes of our relatives.

As we enter the old growth Hemlock Forest, we naturally quiet ourselves. We recognize the extreme gift of communing with these Ancestors. This is a time of prayer and reverence. Eventually I might sing or hum, but first I need to listen and allow myself to align with the vibration of the Forest. Awe requires silence. We might gasp or even laugh at the incredibleness of these Trees. But words dilute the magic.

Silence allows us to absorb the Forest and open our "big ears." We hear the birds and other animals. We hear the wind. We see more as we move slowly and focus on our experience. Our attention and devotion are gifts of reciprocity.

When we hear a sound, we think that it occurred outside of ourselves. The vibration started somewhere else, but the sound (or at least the perception of sound) began inside our ear. The vibration resonates within the cells of our body. The bird songs are a part of us. As the sounds of Nature permeate our body we move into communion, the vibration awakens our sense of belonging. We remember that we are all part of the living Earth; there is no separation.

For most of us, silence is a rare occurrence. By silence, I do not mean the complete absence of sound, which is unsettling, but the absence of man-made noise. Even in wilderness areas, we hear planes flying, maintenance crews with chainsaws, or hunters' gunshots. We are accustomed to noise and don't notice it nor its effects on our body until we experience its absence. But noise disrupts our communion. We add to the noise by listening to music while we are in Nature. While music is wonderful (I love music), too often we utilize music as a distraction from the overwhelm of the noise in our heads. This symptomatic approach interferes with our connection with Nature. We can learn to retrain our thoughts and internal noise so that we do not need distraction and can simply enjoy the silence of Nature. As we listen to Nature, we learn, we heal, and we connect.

I am noise sensitive. I feel the effect the sound of traffic has on my body, ramping up my nervous system. While we can get used to this, it doesn't mean that it no longer affects us. Knowing the effect sound has on me, I wonder about the birds, the Plants, the whales, and our other relatives. There have been numerous studies that show human activity and noise impacts the well-being of animals. Perhaps we prefer the distraction because we are afraid of what we would hear if we listened to our relatives.

Transformation of Death

When I speak to groups, I am often asked what to do for a dying Tree or a Tree that was cut down. People carry great guilt and grief about these deaths. They feel responsible and want to know how to apologize. Sometimes they carry this pain for years. I try to explain that Plants look at death very differently than we do. They understand their role in

Nature. It is helpful to inform a Tree that ki will be cut down and ask if we can do anything for them. It is even better if we ask permission first.

While I have long been aware that Plants look at death differently, Eastern Hemlock gave me a new understanding of this. The first time I was walking in the old growth Forest, I came upon an enormous Hemlock. I could only see the base at first—the trunk was massive. I was awestruck. As I got close to the Tree, I was able to look up. As I did, I reacted and said, "Oh, you're dead." Hemlock quickly responded, "No, I'm not." Ki proceeded to show me all the ways that ki was still alive including mushrooms, lichens, and ants. Hemlock also showed me how ki was feeding and supporting the other Plants nearby. Hemlock said, "Death is not an ending, but a transformation. My life continues in a different form."

Dead standing and even fallen Trees help to shift our understanding of life and a healthy Forest. Mostly, they help us to accept that we do not know as much as we think we know. There is no waste in Nature; every aspect has a purpose and a role and that role contributes to life. Our desire for neat and tidy Landscapes is contrary to Nature and to a healthy ecosystem. The more I work in alignment with Nature, the less work is actually required. I love this! I can leave the dead standing Trees. (Of course, we may need to cut some down if they are at risk of causing harm or for another reason.) I can let the leaves stay on the ground, composting and fertilizing the Land while providing habitat to insects and animals. I mow smaller areas and less frequently. Nature is designed to conserve energy, including my own.

While a Tree may look dead to us, ki is teeming with life. Our society has strict definitions of what is valuable and what is useful. Plants help to shift this. Everything, everyone has value, has something to give, has a place in this beautiful world. It is time that we honor this.

Following Guidance

If we want to work with Nature, we need to be willing to follow guidance. This means understanding that there are Beings who are wiser and have a different perspective than humans. This is part of the purpose of Plant communication. As I said in the beginning, there are numerous gardening and design principles that help us to live in better alignment with Nature. However, most of these are still based on human observation and not actual guidance from Nature. It is easy to fall back into the paradigm of the supremacy of human intelligence. If we want to shift the paradigm, we need to listen to Nature and follow ki's guidance. Of course, if we mess up, we will be presented with another opportunity.

Heart Springs Sanctuary is the first place that I have been able to fully co-create with Nature. Previously I was limited by the expectations of my landlord or my partner. When I moved here, I had the freedom to listen and dream together with Nature. There were a few Plants that I needed to have here for my HEARTransformation classes but almost everything that we did and planted for the first three years was at the direction and request of the Nature Spirits. I really missed having berries, especially Blueberries, so I asked if I could plant Blueberry Bushes. The Nature Spirits agreed and showed me where to plant them. When I shared this with my partner, he said that he thought that Blueberries need more sunlight. I then went back to the Nature Spirits with this information. They showed me another area that was in full sun. In the past, I had amended the soil with Peat Moss for Blueberry Bushes. However, Peat is not a renewable resource and I stopped incorporating ki in my gardening. I asked the Nature Spirits what I could do to help the Blueberries thrive. They showed me how to create a *hügelkultur* bed using the wood from a particular dead standing Tree and augmenting the soil with Pine needles.

I thought that this Tree was a White Pine, which made sense to me since they are acidic. However, when Marcus went to look at the Tree, we discovered that ki was an Eastern Hemlock. Marcus then walked the Sanctuary looking at all of the dead standing Trees. He supposed that the selected Tree was in a place where ki was more likely to provide habitat and that there was another dead standing Eastern Hemlock close to the road and therefore easier to access. Marcus suggested that we cut down this Tree instead and I agreed.

I worked in the garden while Marcus cut down the Tree. Fairly quickly, I noticed that something wasn't right. First, the chain broke on his saw. Marcus fixed it and went back to taking down the Tree. I saw that he was struggling, and the Tree was not falling. I kept checking in and felt that I needed to let Marcus figure this out. He eventually cut the whole way through the trunk and the Tree still would not fall. He wrapped a tow strap around the trunk and tried pulling the Tree over. Nothing happened. Eventually he managed to pull the Tree off of the stump, only to have ki land standing upward. That is when I intervened.

I asked if I could have some time with Eastern Hemlock to see what was happening. The Tree had not fallen over because ki's branches were entwined with those of a Mulberry and a White Pine Tree. When I asked what was going on, all three Trees immediately informed me that we had not asked permission to cut down this Tree, nor was this the Tree that was offered to us, nor had we informed them of our intent. They were stunned. I apologized profusely and asked what they needed and what I could do. They asked for time and gave me suggestions for offerings to make.

I again apologized and shared with Marcus what they told me. He felt horrible. I realized that this was a lesson we needed. We chose human intelligence over Nature's guidance. We needed to remember humility. I needed to be reminded that I can be swayed by the brain and "rational" thinking and I need to trust the guidance that I receive. I also needed to fully learn that a "dead standing" Tree is alive. Sometimes we know things intellectually, but we do not really gnow them bodily. I would never cut down a "living" Tree without first asking and receiving permission. Every cell of my Being now understands that even the rotting wood on the Forest floor is alive and deserves respect and reverence.

We gave our offerings and made amends. The Nature Spirits would not let us look upon ourselves too harshly, though, as that would not have served anyone. We simply needed to acknowledge our mistakes and agree to listen and learn. When I felt that the Trees were ready, I went out to talk with them again. I asked if they were ready to continue and shared what our plans were. They agreed. This time, Marcus barely needed to pull on the tow rope and Eastern Hemlock fell down.

We built the bed using logs and then branches of Eastern Hemlock.

When we were at a farm store, we saw Pine shavings and bought these thinking that they would help to create an acidic soil. We covered the logs with the shavings (instead of the Pine needles) and mixed shavings into the soil, which was piled on top. When we were finished, we planted Blueberry Bushes as well as Thyme and Snapdragons. A couple weeks after planting the Bushes, I read that you do not want to incorporate fresh Pine shavings into gardens because they can take nitrogen away from the Plants—ideally, you let them age for a year or so. Again, we had not followed the guidance, and ultimately the Blueberry Bushes died. However, the Blueberry Bushes planted where the Nature Spirits first showed me continue to thrive.

This year, we added more soil to the hügelkultur bed and planted ki with flowers. We will plant Blueberry Bushes in the bed again next year. From the beginning, we knew that this was an experiment. I didn't realize that part of the experiment would be whether we could follow guidance. We could look at this as a failure or an embarrassment and continue to beat ourselves up. But I prefer to see this as a lesson and a reminder, which I will carry with me whenever I place human intelligence above guidance from the Plants; perhaps you, too, can learn from my lesson. Manulani Aluli Meyer writes, "Kinship with the natural world is about lessons learned to help us awaken."[1] Hemlock is helping me awaken to my role in this beautiful world.

Change with Grace

While I was looking for a Hemlock Tree to connect with, I came to know the Tree through ki's Essence via Kate Gilday, one of my Flower Essence teachers. Kate shared that Eastern Hemlock helps us to move through change with grace. From the beginning of my practice, Eastern Hemlock Essence has been a foundational Essence and one of those most often included in my dosage formulations. Ki continues to support my clients.

Change is an inherent part of life. When we live our lives in accordance with Nature, we learn to embrace and celebrate change. We marvel that we can plant a seed and watch ki sprout and then flower and then fruit all within a few months. In temperate areas, we celebrate the changing colors of autumn. We delight in the migration of birds and butterflies. We understand that there are rhythms of Earth, each connected to the energetic changes that influence the rhythms of our lives. All Indigenous cultures incorporate these rhythms and changes into their cosmology and ceremonies. In the Celtic tradition, there are the High Holy Days (Winter Solstice or Yule, Spring Equinox or Ostara, Summer Solstice or Litha, and Autumn Equinox or Mabon) and the Cross Quarter Days (Imbolc, Beltane, Lammas, Samhain), marking the half-way point between High Holy Days.

Celebrating the rhythms of Nature brings meaning to our lives, reinforcing our connection. But more than that, understanding the rhythms of Nature helps us to know when it is the best time to harvest a food or plant seeds or connect with our Ancestors. When we are in alignment with Nature, we notice the subtle cues (and direct guidance) that help us to know the most auspicious time for something. We don't just know that it is time to celebrate our Ancestors because it is the end of October or the beginning of November. We know it is time because we feel their presence. We know that it is time to tap Maple because the temperature changes—we have warm days and cool nights, and Maple tells us, "It's time."

Incorporating the rhythms of Nature into our lives can seem daunting. There's so much that we don't know and capitalism does not respect the ebb and flow of natural rhythms. However, these rhythms are in our DNA. Everyone has Ancestors who lived in accordance with Nature. For some, these Ancestors are close, and for others they go back many generations. Still, they are there. If this memory feels too distant or lost, well, we are Nature, we can listen to our own bodies. We can try to override the natural rhythms of life, but we cannot escape them. We are them. One of the best ways of healing our connection with Nature is to follow the rhythms. You can start small, maybe by celebrating the Solstices or the shifting Moon phases. Whatever tugs at your Heart, incorporate this into your life. You don't have to be rigid; you also do not need to follow the calendar days (which are often inaccurate); feel the energetic shift in your body, listen to the Plants, the Land, and the water, and move with them.

Because of human activity, many of Earth's rhythms are changing. We see and feel this change. Where I live, flowers that only rarely bloomed for Beltane (May 1) now bloom weeks before. Our first and last frost dates are no longer accurate. It was common for there to be limitations on water usage in August but now we frequently have rain and even flooding then. My friends in California knew that Sacred Springs dried up in November, only to see them dry in July.

The rhythms of Nature are not stagnant. They too change. Usually, though, the change is slower, more gradual. When we are in the midst of such great change it can be easy to become fearful or overwhelmed (as well as to try to become numb and ignore it). It is helpful to remember that the planet has gone through climatic change before. We can look to our more-than-human Ancestors for guidance, especially those Plants who were on the forefront of the great shifts, like Eastern Hemlock. Paw Paw also helps us to navigate the shifting climate. These Plants help us to adapt while staying centered. Being able to adapt and move through change with grace is pivotal to thriving.

Change is an opportunity. We have a tendency to get stuck in our ruts. There is great comfort in routine and patterns. And yet, our routines can lull us into amnesia as we forget innocent perception and limit our growth and evolution. Change encourages creativity and puts us back into the flow of Nature. Change brings excitement and energy.

We often say that we want change. We are frustrated with a situation or feel stagnation, yet when we are presented with an opportunity for change, we run or hide, preferring the known for the unknown. Sometimes we respond to change through our trauma response. We can dive deep into depression or numb ourselves or we can swing the other way and try to take control of the situation (and everyone involved), living off of drama and adrenaline.

For the first few years of my healing practice, I wondered if I should have a disclaimer: "Warning, working with Brigid's Way may lead to job loss or divorce." Almost everyone who I worked with those beginning years ended up leaving or losing their job or ending their significant relationship. They all were happy with the results, knowing that this was necessary for their Soul. However, I felt a bit like Typhoid Mary. Now that my practice has expanded, my clients come to me for many different reasons; some still end up leaving or losing their jobs or ending relationships, but not all.

Large changes like these can leave us disoriented. Our identity has been greatly connected to our job or our relationship. We need to rediscover who we are or even what brings us joy. This loss of identity can frighten us and contribute to the trauma response. Or we can approach it with great gratitude for our ability to re-member who we are and recreate our life to be in alignment with our Soul. To do this, we need a strong root chakra and feeling of safety. Eastern Hemlock supports this. Ki reminds us that we are safe, strengthening our root chakra and connection with the Earth while gently guiding us through change.

When we consciously choose change in order to live the life of our Heart's longing, sometimes those close to us struggle. They may suddenly withdraw or try to talk us out of it. This is not anything personal. Our change affects them and may trigger their own trauma or fear. It may bring to light the areas of their life that are not fulfilling. It can be frightening to change. We can think that the world is ending and the sky is falling. I can assure you that that is not the case, for the world continues to exist. While it can be hard to let go of friends and family while we navigate change, I have witnessed that if we are living our Soul's calling, we will attract people who support our growth and evolution.

At this point in time, we all need to make changes. We cannot continue to live as we have been doing. The shutdowns from COVID showed us how quickly we can change our lives and how quickly Nature can recover and respond to our changes. (As well as, how quickly we want to return to "normal" and how resistant we are to change.) While there is not one thing that we all have to change, such as everyone using solar power or driving an electric car, we do need to listen to our Hearts, our Souls, and our more-than-human relatives. How are you being asked to change?

Indigenous cultures know to celebrate and honor the great thresholds of life. There is an understanding that everyone and everything changes, and change helps us to evolve and expand our consciousness. The eco-society of Damanhur in Italy recognizes the power of change. When there is conflict or stagnation within the community, they require people to change their jobs and/or their homes. Even outside of these times, it is encouraged that community members frequently change jobs, understanding that these changes promote growth and stability for the individual and the community.

Often those who struggle the most with change experienced great trauma as a child. They never knew what they could rely on. They long for stability. It is a little ironic, because maintaining the status quo does not promote stability. Stability occurs through flexibility and adaptability.

Darwin's theory of evolution and the resulting belief in the survival of the fittest has greatly impacted our experience of the world including our response to change. Unfortunately, this theory was written through the lens of aristocracy and was used to give credence to some being superior to others. The full title of his famous book is *On the Origin of Species by Means of Natural Selection, or the Preservation of Favoured Races in the Struggle for Life*. His theory has been interpreted that only the strongest survive, thus supporting competition and ruthlessness. In fact, evolution shows us that those who survive are those most able to adapt. As Bruce Lipton says it is not survival of the fittest, but the "thrival of the fittingest."[2] Adaptability leads to thriving.

Survival of the fittest encourages us to rape the Earth, taking what we can, focusing only on our own desires. It imposes a hierarchy and a global contest for King of the Mountain. Whereas, thrival of the fittingest reminds us of the necessity of relationship and community. It brings us back into the circle with all life. Thrival of the fittingest encourages cooperation and adaptation which is exactly the model that Plants provide. To thrive, we change with grace.

Flower Essences

Flower Essences are the energetic imprint of a Plant captured in water and preserved with another substance, usually brandy. This is the definition that I most often give for a Flower Essence, but I could just as easily define Flower Essences as agents of change.

Flower Essences focus on the root cause of a situation. Sometimes people contact me because they get frequent headaches and ask what Essence I recommend. This is not how they work. The headache is a symptom. We need to know what is behind the headache. Is it tension? Is there a lack of sleep? Is this connected to something from childhood? Are they perfectionists? Are they ungrounded? Are they holding on to traumas? Flower Essences shift our vibration, providing an opportunity to experience life differently. Dr. Edward Bach, the originator of modern-day Flower Essences, wrote, "Thus, behind all disease lie our fears, our anxieties, our greed, our likes and dislikes. Let us seek these out and heal them, and with the healing of them will go the disease from which we suffer."[3]

Flower Essences help to remove the energetic imprints from the traumas, fears, beliefs, and blocks that are inhibiting the body's innate healing ability. They give us a reprieve allowing us to remember our Truth. They may also bring forward aspects of our subconscious that we have suppressed. Because of this, it is helpful to work with a practitioner, especially when focusing on deep healing work. Flower Essences are often referred to as subtle and gentle. This can be true, but it is not the full truth. Essences can be incredibly potent. Some Essences are too strong for certain people; they can bring up something that someone is not ready for or doesn't have the support system to work through. A good practitioner is aware of this.

As part of a recent class, I worked with Wood Lily Essence. Wood Lily helps with repressed anger. I have worked with this Essence for over ten years, occasionally giving ki to my clients. Even so, I was not prepared for the rollercoaster I experienced with Wood Lily. Old, repressed memories resurfaced. I felt a level of anger I never had access to. Fortunately for my Beloved, I knew that this anger was old and I had tools for processing it rather than projecting it. I really appreciate the healing gifts I received from Wood Lily Essence and there is a good reason I only include this Essence in a blend with supportive Essences for my clients.

It may seem odd that something that physically is simply water and brandy could elicit a strong effect. We need to remember that Essences are energetic in Nature and there is much more to our world than what we generally accept. We know that Flower Essences work because we can witness the changes. Sometimes, though, if we are the one experiencing the change, we may not notice it. We get used to our current situation, akin to the frog in the pot, so it is helpful to have someone else who can remind us of what life was like before taking the Essence.

Since Dr. Bach's time, the world of Flower Essences has greatly blossomed. There are Essences made with Plants from all over the world. These Essences are not only made with flowers, but also Trees, mushrooms, gems, environments, animals, other worldly Beings, and more. I see this vast array of Essences as a sign of Nature's Love for us and conspiracy to help us to heal and re-member. One of the benefits of Essences is that they require little to no physical material to make. Therefore we can avoid over harvesting and work with rare and poisonous Plants. These little bottles give us access to Plants and places we would not otherwise have access to. When you experience an Essence that is right for you, there is a realization that you are loved and held by Nature. We are encouraged to remember who we are and to release the burdens and untruths that we have been carrying.

Besides helping with our healing and evolution, Essences are a wonderful way of getting to know a Plant. They are inexpensive, easy to transport, and, if stored properly, last a long time (like a lifetime). Flower Essences are often confused with Essential Oils. Again, Essences are the energetic imprint of a Plant. They contain little to no physical Plant material in them and thus they do not have a smell. Essential Oils contain the volatile aromatic principles of Plants (or the chemicals that contribute to a Plant's smell) and utilize these for healing. A large amount of a Plant is required to produce a small amount of Essential Oil. Many Essential Oils are toxic if they are ingested. Essences and Essential Oils are quite different.

Different practitioners utilize different methods for making Essences. Some go to great lengths to keep their energy out of the Essence. Essences are energetic preparations; it is impossible to remove one's energy from their creation. Moreover, the human is an essential part of the Essence.

An Essence represents the alchemical relationship between the human, Plant (or other Being), and water. Therefore, Essences of the same Plant made by different people will have a similar core theme and will be energetically different. There will be some companies whose Essences you resonate with and others you don't—trust this instinct.

Since I work with Plant and Nature Spirits, I invite the Spirit of the Plant to be part of the Essence. Therefore, I refer to my Essences as Spirit Essences. (Many of mine are also made with aspects of Nature other than flowers.) Not all Essences contain the Spirit of the Plant. I feel this makes a difference. Including the Spirit of the Plant creates a more complete form of the Plant's Essence and gifts.

When making Essences, I wait for a Plant to call me; after all, this is about relationship. Sometimes there will be a Plant that I want to make an Essence with. I express my desire and wait for an invitation. I then follow the Plant's guidance in the making of the Essence. Traditionally an Essence is made in the sun for two hours. But we are working on an energetic level, so not every Essence requires two hours; some are immediate, some want to be created over a longer period, some Essences prefer to be made with the moon, and some like a combination of sun and moon.

The quality of water is critical to making an Essence. You want to use the purest water possible. Definitely do not use chlorinated tap water. Some people are particular about the bowl. I use a clear glass bowl from Crate and Barrel. This is what David Dalton gave us in our training and I have continued to use the same kind ever since. I have made a few Essences in special bowls, including ones made from stone, but clear glass works great.

When I get the message that it is time to create an Essence, I fill my bowl halfway with water. I take this outside and place ki near the Plant. I say prayers with the Plant and invite the Spirit of the Plant to fill this bowl, allowing the water to carry ki's imprint and healing gifts. I also ask for guidance in the creation and utilization of the Essence. Then I follow the Plant's request. Sometimes I sit with the Plant. Sometimes I sing. Sometimes I leave the Plant alone until I get the message that the Essence is complete.

I no longer include physical Plant parts in my Essences, unless the Plant adds them. I learned that we do not need to include the physical components when we make Essences with rare or poisonous Plants. Therefore, I realized I would not need to include them for any other Essence. Many of my Essences are made when I'm traveling. I often do not know if a Plant is poisonous; sometimes I do not even know the name of the Plant. To be safe, I stopped including the physical Plant with no decrease in efficacy. After all, these are energetic preparations.

When the Essence is complete, I bring a two-ounce bottle that is partially filled with brandy to the Plant (I use a ratio of 40 percent brandy to 60 percent Essence water). I then fill the bottle the rest of the way with the Essence water. If any insects or Plant parts fell into the water, I make sure that they are not in the bottle, straining if necessary. This creation is called the Mother Essence. I label this bottle including when and where I made the Essence.

Flower Essences, like homeopathy, use a dilution method. The Mother Essence, which is made directly from the Plant, is diluted to create the Stock Essence. The Stock Essence is what you buy at a store. We make the Stock by filling a half-ounce bottle with 40 percent brandy and 60 percent water (again you want the purest water available). We then add 3 drops of the Mother Essence into this bottle. The Stock Essence is more aligned with physical issues. I work with them using a technique that was developed by David Dalton to help shift the energetic patterns of physical ailments. I also work with the Stock for journeying and dreaming with an Essence, taking one drop of the Stock before the journey.

Most of the time we ingest a Dosage Essence. If you work with a Flower Essence practitioner, this is what they create for you. To make a Dosage Essence we fill a half-ounce bottle with 30 percent brandy and 70 percent water. To this bottle, we add three drops of the Stock Essence. A Dosage Essence is aligned more with our emotional and spiritual bodies. Please know that we can still experience physical healing by ingesting a Dosage Essence, since physical ailments generally begin with disturbances in the emotional and spiritual bodies. Generally, we take a Dosage Essence for a set period of time, usually about a month. The typical suggested dosage is three drops, three times a day. We can either place these directly in our mouth, under the tongue (being very careful not to touch the dropper to our mouth) or place them in water or another beverage. If you follow this dosage, you will finish a half-ounce bottle in about a month.

We can combine several Essences in the Dosage Essence. Most of the time, a Flower Essence practitioner formulates a blend specifically for you. We do this by adding three drops of each chosen Stock Essence (though the amount can vary) into the Dosage bottle.

One of the issues with Essences is the alcohol preservative. Some companies use Shiso vinegar instead of alcohol, which has a shorter shelf life. I use water as the base for the Dosage bottle if I know that my client will complete the bottle within a month. While Essences contain significantly less alcohol than a tincture or cough syrup, they do taste like brandy. If the taste of alcohol is a trigger for you, you can add the Essences to your juice or tea. If you prefer to avoid alcohol consumption, you can put the Essences on your body. Placing them on acupuncture points can be extremely effective. If you are energetically sensitive, you can hold the bottle and meditate or have the bottle next to you as you sleep.

After making an Essence, we want to "test" ki to discover the healing gifts of this Essence. We do that by taking a drop of the Stock and journeying with ki. Or taking a drop of the Stock before bed. We also take the Dosage Essence for at least a week, ideally a month, noticing any shifts. We can ask others to take the Essence, helping to broaden our understanding of the Essence and confirm the core gifts.

In my apprenticeship, I give everyone a drop of an Essence. After sitting for about ten minutes, I ask what they noticed. Or other times we do a journey with an Essence and share our experiences. Through these processes, we begin to see a common experience. It is also a way for my students to have a body memory of an Essence and to strengthen their ability to sense energy. When they learn how to make an Essence, they make bottles to share with their classmates. Everyone is given an unlabeled bottle to test for a month. I compile their experiences and share them with the group. It is amazing to see the similar threads for each Essence even when they didn't know what Plant they were working with.

While there is so much to say and learn about Essences, the reason for including them in this book is that they are a wonderful way of getting to know your Plant ally. Essences can help to open us up to a different world.

Exercise: Making an Essence with Your Plant Ally

Having an Essence of your Plant gives you easy access to ki, allowing you to carry the Plant with you at all times and experience ki in a different way. Making an Essence is a special experience, another way of connecting. In the end, you have an alchemical Essence that represents your unique relationship with your Plant ally. Plus, you can receive other guidance and insight as you make and test the Essence.

- Gather the supplies that you need for making your Essence: a thin glass bowl or other vessel, pure water (not chlorinated), brandy or other preservative, clean bottles, and labels. I use a two-ounce bottle (with dropper) for my Mother Essences and half-ounce bottles (with dropper) for the Stock and Dosage Essences. Most health food stores and herbalists sell these bottles. Because I sell my Essences, I do not reuse bottles, but if this is for your own use, you may have a bottle you can repurpose. Be sure that you sterilize any clean, reused bottles in boiling water.

- While gathering your supplies, connect with your Plant ally and let them know that you would like to make an Essence with them. Ask them to inform you of the best time to do this.

- When the time is right, fill your bowl with water. Place this near or on the Plant. Decide if you are going to place Plant parts into the bowl and if so, collect these with permission and prayer.

- Connect with your Plant ally. Say prayers for the creation of this Essence, asking the Plant to pour their energy and, if you like, Spirit, into the bowl, allowing the water to carry the imprint of them. Ask for guidance on the creation and usage of this Essence. Follow the Plant's direction.

When the Essence is complete, fill your Mother Essence bottle 40 percent full with brandy. (If using a two-ounce bottle this is .8 ounces.) Then pour enough Essence water into this bottle to fill it completely. Be sure that no Plant material or debris entered the bottle. If they did, strain them out. Label this bottle as the Mother Essence of your Plant.

- You most likely have Essence water left. I like to take a small sip of this and then gift the rest to the Plant. Of course, offer your gratitude.
- Make a Stock bottle from your Mother Essence. Fill a half-ounce bottle with a mixture of 40 percent brandy and 60 percent water, and add three drops of the Mother Essence into this bottle. Be sure to label this bottle as well, including that this is the Stock Essence.
- Now it's time to test and experience the Essence. Take one drop of the Stock Essence and do a journey. On another day, take a drop of the Stock before bed or take a drop of the Stock and lay down for a nap. Write down your experiences, paying attention to your dreams and how you felt both during the journey or sleep and upon waking.
- When you are ready, make a Dosage Essence. Fill a half-ounce bottle with 30 percent brandy and 70 percent water or use a base of 100 percent water (just be sure to finish this within a month or gift the remaining Dosage Essence to the Plants). To this bottle, add 3 drops of the Stock Essence. Again, standard dosage for an Essence is to take three drops three times a day for a month. Notice any differences in your body, your emotions, your perceptions. Did you receive any information from your Plant ally? How did it feel to take ki's Essence several times a day? Could you feel ki supporting you?
- If you are able to, you may want to share your Essence with friends and collect their experiences.

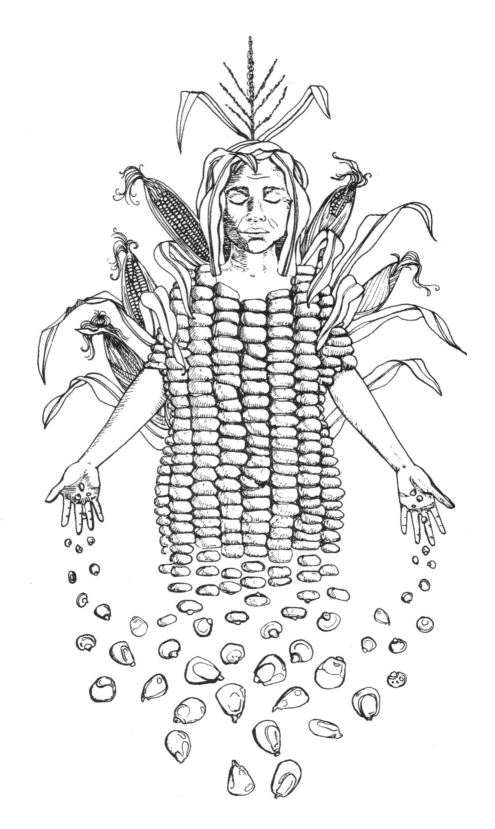

15
❧ The Great Mother ❧
Corn

Growing up in Lancaster County, Pennsylvania, Corn has been a significant part of my life. Lancaster County is known for having "some of the most fertile non-irrigated land in the country."[1] The two most prized vegetables are Tomatoes and Corn. Everyone looked forward to Sweet Corn, which usually was available around the beginning of August or, if we were lucky, the end of July. We celebrated Corn season with a ravenous gluttony, slathering the ears with butter and salt. This was our manna from heaven. Silver Queen was the preferred variety, ki's small, white kernels bursting with sweetness, a perfect match for butter and salt. The three main seasonings of Pennsylvania Dutch cooking are butter, salt, and sugar (in this case in the form of sugar enhanced Corn).

My grandfather grew his own Corn, which he brought to our family gatherings. I would help him shuck, and inevitably would shriek in surprise because his Corn always had earworms. My grandfather would say, "They don't eat much! It's extra protein." He'd leave the earworms; I tried to find a way to secretly get rid of them. Still, his Corn was my favorite.

During the growing season, we ate as much Corn as possible to sustain us through the year. Many families gathered together to freeze bushels of Corn. Everyone knew that the best frozen Corn could not be found in a store; one of the most treasured gifts you could receive was plastic pouches of frozen Lancaster County Corn. While my parents did not partake in this ritual, both sets of grandparents did. Our holiday tables were graced with bowls of Corn, of course shimmering with butter, and occasionally we were treated to my Nanny's delicious Chicken Corn Soup.

It is interesting to me that as I look back, no one seemed to think it strange that Corn was a pivotal component of Pennsylvania Dutch cooking. Nor did they question the relationship between Corn and German immigrants. We simply celebrated Corn as part of our heritage without understanding what this meant. I'm sure at one point we were told that Native Americans introduced Corn to our Ancestors, most likely shared as part of the giant lie about the Thanksgiving feast. According to Michael Pollan, "Squanto taught the Pilgrims how to plant maize in the spring of 1621, and the colonists immediately recognized its value: No other plant could produce quite as much food quite as fast on a given patch of New World ground as this Indian corn."[2] Did the pilgrims share the knowledge of Corn with the other colonists or did the German immigrants learn from the Susquehannocks and Lenni Lenape who lived here? I guess it is common to not know the origins of our food; however, this is another way of wiping out Indigenous knowledge, feeding into the "savage" myth. Ironically the survival of the immigrants and the nation that they created was due to the superior wisdom of these "savages."

It is generally believed that Corn evolved from Teosinte in what we now call Mexico. I have heard accounts that this evolution occurred seven to ten thousand years ago. Some scientists claim that this was a natural form of evolution, while others state that the Indigenous peoples bred and selected the Plants to create a more edible form that evolved into Corn. One of the great gifts of Corn is the ability to adapt and respond to the environment and people. It is this adaptability that has led to the enormous number of varieties of Corn and the many different colors, shapes, and sizes. Again, scientists are trying to understand how Corn has evolved and spread through the Americas and they often get stumped. Though to me it seems obvious: Corn has a deep intimate connection with the people who grow ki. There is no separation, or at least once upon a time there wasn't. This is why each Indigenous group in a certain area had their unique, Sacred Corn varieties.

Co-evolution of People and Plants

Plants have always evolved before their animal counterparts, especially Humans. It is their evolution that has led to our creation. We witness the intimacy of our co-evolution through the beautiful relationship of Orchids and pollinators. *Angraecum sesquipedale,* or Darwin's Orchid, is an exquisite example. This Orchid is endemic to Madagascar and has a nectary almost a foot long. Darwin theorized that there must be a moth with a tongue just as long. Almost 150 years later, scientists confirmed such a moth in Madagascar.

As our Ancestors moved through the world, they brought their seeds with them. There are numerous accounts of African women braiding seeds into their hair in case they were kidnapped and taken to foreign Lands. While we can romanticize these stories, elevating the poetic, the truth is that these were acts of desperation and survival. Seeds allowed our Ancestors to bring Home with them, but even more than that, they held the promise of nourishment and future generations. For our Ancestors, seeds were often the most Sacred Beings, providing hope and life, anchors during a time of uncertainty and trauma.

Thus seeds migrated to new Lands with the people they nourished. The Plants of these seeds intermingled with the Plants of seeds from other Lands. People shared their foods and seeds with one another. The seeds were transformed and shaped by the different soils and rains and weather. New breeds were created. Some flourished and some perished. Our Ancestors helped to form the Plants. While they ate these new foods, the Plants helped to form them. We talk about Darwin and evolution as if this occurred a long time ago and is now complete. But we continue to evolve and shape one another.

In our modern culture, we forget the preciousness of seeds. Grocery stores offer us an abundance of food throughout the year. We do not have to preserve our food or grow fruits and vegetables who store well. We no longer need to save or carry our seeds with us. There are seed companies and catalogs with lush and beautiful images. We can order these seeds from anywhere. Those who remain close to the Land know that growing and preserving your own food is the ultimate source of nourishment (on all levels), even if you have one Tomato Plant or one Basil Plant. The Plants are formed by their relationship with us. They adapt to the Land where we live, and they provide what we need more than the most beautiful vegetable in any store.

COVID was a great reminder of the importance of growing your own food, which requires seeds. Despite the grocery stores and the plethora of catalogues, what was true for our Ancestors remains true for us: our lives are dependent on seeds.

Rocío Alarcón deepened my relationship with seeds. In our training, we were taught that seeds are healers and protectors, that they carry the potential. We wear seeds, we make sound with seeds, and we create Healing Landscapes (similar to an altar) with seeds. Thanks to this work, I have a cabinet filled with jars of seeds. I did save a few seeds prior to this training, but now, seeds have rooted in my Being. I gather them. I am gifted them. I stare at them. I feel them. I am mesmerized by their incredible shapes and sizes and colors. I wonder about their story, who held them before, who planted them, who loved them? It astonishes me that whole Plants or even Trees come from these tiny packets.

My collection is beginning to become unwieldy, and therefore my gathering has slowed, though sometimes it's difficult to restrain myself. These seeds are prayers. When I or someone I know, be they a friend or client, needs support, I turn to the cabinet of seeds. Together we create a prayer. The seeds who come forward help me to understand the energetics of the issue. These seeds from around the world are continuing to form me. As my sisters would say, "I am one seedy woman."

I admit that as much as I am a seed saver, when it comes to the garden, I often turn to the support of the seed catalogs. Nowadays this is often about convenience and time. But it used to be because I didn't trust my ability to save seeds. I greatly appreciated Leah Penniman sharing her own hesitation in *Farming While Black*:

Even after a decade of farming, I was intimidated by the idea of saving seed. I imagined that the people who packed seeds into those tiny paper envelopes and mailed them to me each year had some secret inaccessible magic to make those seeds viable. I did not trust myself not to ruin the life force potential of these tiny beings of possibility. I did not trust the plants growing on my farm to make progeny as healthy and vibrant as those I could purchase in the store. Of course, I realize that I had internalized the corporate messaging of agricultural megacorporations, which try to get us to believe that we are not good enough to steward our genetic heritage. I was wrong.[3]

Gathering and saving seeds is another way to awaken our innate connection with Nature. We may feel clumsy at first, but as we begin, our DNA stirs. When we grow a Plant from seeds that we saved or were gifted to us, we step further into our role as co-creators. Not to mention we feel like kickass superheroes.

Saving seeds is a way of celebrating, as Leah states, "our genetic heritage," but more than that, saving and sharing our seeds is economical. It is an insurance policy, making it more likely that we will have food next year. Sadly, with industrial agriculture, our seed diversity is diminishing. There are more and more organizations who are focused on saving our heritage seeds, knowing that our future may very well depend on them. But as Martín Prechtel writes, "It is not enough to save heritage seeds. The culture of those people to whom each seed belongs must be kept alive along with seeds and their cultivation. Not in freezers or museums but in their own soil and our daily lives."[4]

One of the biggest issues concerning seeds is the emphasis on Genetically Modified (or GMO) seeds, which companies can own and patent. There are many arguments for and against GMOs. My answer is to ask the Plants. From my experience, GMO Plants do not feel vibrant, they don't carry the life force or the spark that Plants traditionally have. Perhaps it is because they are created to withstand being sprayed by poisons. As Vandana Shiva writes, "Whatever happens to seed affects the web of life."[5] These seeds are our genetic heritage; do we want them to be poisoned? If so, what genetic heritage do we leave for our future generations? Are we going to remember the Sacred gift of a seed?

Corn People

In my seed cabinet, there are several varieties of Corn. I have Flint Popcorn, Red Corn, Blue Corn, a large kernel yellow Corn, Glass Gem Corn, a multicolored Corn, and Birth/Death Corn (which I grow). Birth/Death Corn comes from the Tz'utujil Mayan in Guatemala via Martín Prechtel. Martín shares the extraordinary story of this Corn and the Tz'utujil in his beautiful book *The Unlikely Peace at Cuchumaquic: The Parallel Lives of People as Plants: Keeping the Seeds Alive.* This Corn is part of the birth and death rituals of the Tz'utujil. It is through ki that life continues, allowing the Tz'utujil to become seeds to sprout again. It is hard for the domesticated to understand the deep intimacy and interconnectedness of the Tz'utujil Mayan and this Corn. Martín writes, "Ethnologists might say the villagers and corn had parallel lives, but the reality of it was for the Tzutujil that corn and the people were right and left halves of the same organism, and that organism lived by the principles of seeds as maintained ritually by both halves to keep it whole."[6] This is not a symbolic relationship. The Tz'utujil Mayan are Corn.

The same can be said for other Indigenous peoples—they, too, consider themselves Corn People. Corn provided the sustenance of life, both physically and spiritually. For many, Corn is the Great Mother who birthed them into being. Taíno farmers called this Plant "mahiz," meaning "source of life."[7]

For me, this Sacred Birth/Death Corn is the epitome of resilience and hope. There is no reason why a White woman in Pennsylvania should be growing this Corn. Ki was not grown for daily consumption. This is ceremonial Corn. I have no connection to the ceremonies of the Tz'utujil, I've never been to Guatemala. Yet, for the past seven years I have been growing this Corn and this Corn has been growing me.

Birth/Death Corn found ki's way to me through trauma and violence and an insatiable responsibility to carry forth life. For decades, the people, especially the Indigenous, of Guatemala were subjected to horrific violence and destruction due to the United States-backed regimes. These regimes used a tactic from the old colonialism playbook: when you want to control someone, you take away their food. In an act of revenge, they scorched the fields and mountains of Guatemala, including where the Tz'utujil lived. The Birth/Death Corn disappeared.

But life does not give up so easily, and miraculously this Corn once again ended up in the hands of Martín Prechtel. (You'll have to read his book to truly grasp the miracle of this precious Corn.) Martín shares his Corn with his students and has discovered that the Corn changes color and form depending on who grows ki. But of course, Corn adapts to the environment and people where ki grows. Scientists can argue that this is because Corn is wind-pollinated, but this is the interrelationship between Corn and People.

Martín gifted Pam Montgomery and Mark Carlin with seeds. They grew this Corn for many years and gifted me three Birth/Death Corn seeds during my Plant Spirit Healing Apprenticeship. I was enamored with this Corn and felt the responsibility of ki's survival as well as doubt in my ability to properly grow ki, partially because there was a large field of GMO Corn next to our farm. I was concerned about cross-pollination. How could I grow this Corn in an honorable way?

At the time, my healing office was in our strawbale house, as we built and moved into our "big house." I placed these three seeds in a beautiful bowl and set them on my altar. I thought that I could honor them best by praying with them. The resident mice quickly discovered my offering and were grateful for my generosity, eating all three seeds. I was heartbroken and ashamed. I knew that I could ask Pam for more seeds, but I was too ashamed to admit my disrespect.

Several years later, I was gifted three Birth/Death Corn seeds by my friends Tammi and Kris. They too had received their original seeds from Pam and Mark. This time I knew that Corn needed to be in the ground, not on a shelf or in a cabinet. Fortunately, I had moved from the farm and did not have any Cornfields nearby. If you know anything about growing Corn, ki likes to grow in a large patch; normally you plant hundreds or thousands of seeds, not three. Miraculously, all three seeds sprouted and produced the most beautiful, perfect white ear of Corn.

I have continued to grow this Corn every year. I once again have neighboring Cornfields. Fortunately, there is a push to plant Corn as quickly as possible. The Sweet Corn of my childhood, which was "knee high by the fourth of July" and available in August, is now available on the fourth of July. I try to protect the genetics of Birth/Death Corn by planting ki long after the field Corn is planted. One year, I planted Corn in a new garden bed. Ki sprouted, growing very tall. One day we had an enormous storm with high winds whip through the Sanctuary. The Cornstalks were knocked over, some even uprooted. I planted the roots again and all survived, though they were horizontal. But not for long. Soon, the tops of the Corn continued to grow straight up, creating interesting angles in the stalks. Once again, Corn demonstrated ki's resiliency and the ability to stand tall in one's Being, no matter what knocks you down.

Every year, I gift three kernels of Birth/Death Corn to my students. I also grind this Corn to give as offerings, using a hand crank grain mill. As I grind, I sing and say prayers. I remember the remarkable journey of this Corn and I give gratitude for the Tz'utujil. I don't know that I will ever see their Lands or meet a Tz'utujil in person, but I hope that my tending and honoring of this Corn feeds them. It is a small act of gratitude to them for keeping the memory alive. As I engage with Birth/Death Corn, I can feel ki gently tugging me back into kinship.

I do not refer to this Corn as Birth/Death Corn. I simply call ki Grandmother. This is not symbolic. A grandmother surrounds her grandchild with Love. A grandmother sees the potential of the child and holds that image for them, gently coaxing when they have lost their way. A grandmother shares the family stories, helping the child to discover their place in this world. As the child grows, they understand that they are responsible for the care of their grandmother. It is their turn to shower their relative with Love, reinforcing her role in the family and this world. *Grand* refers to magnificent and great. Thus, I call this Corn Grandmother.

Prayer

My preference is to grow Grandmother Corn next to our deck. I like to listen to the wind in ki's leaves. I noticed that Grandmother also enjoys this location. When my students are here, ki leans toward the deck, pushing through the railing. Grandmother wants to be in relationship with us, to be part of our circle and meals.

When I began to grow Grandmother Corn, I was aware that the Tz'utujil held ceremonies throughout the growing and processing period. This Corn was bathed in prayers and Love. I did not know these ceremonies or prayers; how could I honor this Sacred Corn?

Prayer and I had a difficult relationship. For the first four years of my schooling, I attended a fundamental Christian school. We were taught that we needed to pray for our sins. I remember driving with my mom, covering my ears and begging her to change the radio station because I was told that rock and roll was the devil's music. I was convinced that I was going to hell for listening to it. In high school, I was involved in our local AIDS project. I remember times when I was followed by a group of people praying for my Soul because I associated with the gay community.

Prayer did not feel nourishing to me. It felt like a reminder of my unworthiness. It was oppressive and controlling. Because of this, I turned my back on prayer for a long time. I would get upset when some- one would say that they were praying for me; I didn't want their prayers. I wanted them to keep their God and judgment to themselves.

It took me years to soften to the understanding that prayer is not owned by fundamental Christians. It is not meant to be a tool of control and oppression. Prayer is a conversation with Spirit. It is a way to share our intentions for this world and honor the incredible Beings who bless our lives and this Earth. Through prayer, we speak our Heart's desires, be they world peace, healing for a friend, clean water, Love, guidance, or gratitude. When we speak, our words carry a vibration that affects the air around us, rippling out. This vibration gives form to what is in our Heart. We speak with honesty, humility, and sweetness. Our words feed the Spirits, helping to create the world.

Prayer is more than words spoken. Our lives are prayers. When I walk barefoot on Earth, I can consciously send my Love and gratitude through my feet, kissing the Earth as I walk. When I cook, I can fill the food with my Love and prayers for my family or students. There are so many ways in which we can pray, and none of them require that you be on your knees, hands clasped and head bowed. We can pray through making Love, reading to a child, tending to a friend who is ill, or building a house. There is no limit. We only need to hold the intention and be aligned with Love.

Prayer, which I once shunned, is now an integral part of my life. I embrace prayer in all forms. I routinely light candles and say prayers for friends who are ill or experiencing difficulties. I ask others to pray for me during my own challenges. I no longer turn my back on receiving prayers. It doesn't matter to me who they are praying to because I know that ultimately, they are simply adding energy to my own conversation with Spirit. And I choose to see the Love in their words.

Singing to Plants

My grandfather taught me to sing to the Plants. He played classical music in his greenhouse. We sang in the garden. My grandmother has a habit of humming throughout her day. I'm not sure if she is even aware of it. I too hum as I'm cooking or driving or simply moving about the house. I discovered that I hummed whenever I spent time in Nature, especially if I was alone. It seemed natural to me. I would walk or sit with a Plant and a song would emerge. As I became conscious of this, I started to notice the reaction of the Land and Plants. I saw that my song could help to heal or strengthen or uplift the area. One day, I woke with the gnowing that I needed to sing the world awake. I greeted each morning with the song of the Land. Later I discovered Terry Tempest Williams's beautiful quote, "Once upon a time, when women were birds, there was the simple understanding that to sing at dawn and to sing at dusk was to heal the world through joy."[8] Singing reflects the longing of our Soul to be in relationship with Nature. As we sing, the world responds, whether we are aware of this or not. After all, we are part of the uni-verse, or "one song." As the people in Damanhur say, there once was one song, one frequency—but then, humans separated. Singing helps us to repair this separation.

Since I don't know the prayers or ceremonies for the Birth/Death Corn, I improvise. Before planting, I place each seed in my mouth. I water them with my body, surrounding them with my Love. I gently place the seed in Earth, speaking prayers of gratitude and prayers for their nourishment and growth. Each day I look for the miraculous green shoots of life. As I wait, I sing to the seeds buried in the Earth. I hope my voice will encourage them to grow. When they appear, I hoot with delight. I praise their bravery and strength. I sing prayers telling them of their exquisite beauty. I try to visit Grandmother every morning and sing to ki. I send energetic prayers of Love. I am in awe of ki's growth. I swear you can watch Corn grow every day. When Grandmother's flowers form and the tassels appear, I celebrate often with song and tears of joy. Sometimes I dance my prayers with Grandmother. At least, this is what I generally do.

Like everyone else, 2020 was a challenging year for me. Though my experience seemed to be quite different, from what I saw on the news. I did not have more time on my hands. I was not able to focus on cleaning my house or baking bread and I definitely wasn't bored. I already worked from home and Marcus had just started going into his office the week before lockdown. So we quickly adjusted to both of us working here. I planned to teach both levels of the HEARTransformation Apprenticeship. I considered canceling, but when I checked in, I heard that it was important to offer this work at this time. These classes are designed to occur in person. We tried to delay them hoping that the pandemic would end quickly, which did not happen. Therefore, I had to completely rework the advanced program and greatly readjust the first-year program. Suddenly, my workload doubled and then tripled as we tried to navigate the emotions and needs of my students and create a healthy place to gather. The enormous time and energetic commitment required that I let go of other activities. It wasn't until months into the growing season that I realized I stopped singing to Grandmother. I was reminded when I saw ki flowering. I couldn't remember the last time that I had sung or greeted ki, even though Grandmother was right next to our porch.

I was wracked with guilt. But it seemed that Grandmother had a lesson to teach. When I harvested ki, I was shocked at the ears of Corn. There were very few ears, and most of them were completely rotten or had only a few kernels on them. None of these ears contained the pure white Corn I grew before. The deformed ears served as a physical reminder of the importance of singing and praying. Hopefully, I will never again forget my role in the growing of Grandmother Corn.

Yes, Plants enjoy when we sing to them. But of course, birds and other animals sing to them. The buzzing of a bumblebee makes the sound of middle C and causes flowers to release more pollen. Sound is a key component to communication. While we rarely hear a Bush booming a message for us, we still incorporate sound into our communication process. So far, we have been listening with our intuition. We also sing or perhaps play instruments for our Plant ally. As we do, we pay attention to how the Plant responds. Is there a particular sound or rhythm that they enjoy? What sounds naturally emerge as we connect with the Plant? What do these sounds evoke in us? Listening with your mind's eye, is there a tune or song that the Plant is sharing?

A vibration occurs as we sing. This vibration is affected by our Plant ally. As our bodies resonate with the song of our Plant, we bathe our cells in this energy. We may notice sensations or messages emerging. We want to pay attention to these as they are part of our Plant ally's story.

When we get to the sound component of a Plant communication weekend, people often get self-conscious. Many of us have been told that we are not good singers. This is a horrible thing to say to someone, especially a child. We may not all be Adele, but our voices are meant to be expressed. Plants are not interested in critiquing your singing ability. They hear the energy and intent behind the notes. Singing from the Heart is another way to share your prayer and Love with the world. Ideally, we sing with our whole body, letting our prayer pour forth. Despite my music teacher's admonishments, I have never had a Plant recoil from my song, or complain or ask me to stop. Instead, they often encourage me to sing more.

Music of the Plants

We not only sing to the Plants; now we can hear the Plants sing to us, thanks to the creation of an instrument called the Music of the Plants device. This device was created in the late 1970s in the eco-society of Damanhur. The intention was to demonstrate that Plants are intelligent and to help humans deepen their connection with the Plant world.

I have worked with the Music of the Plants since 2013 and became their first distributor in 2014. It is a gift to share this instrument with others. Frequently, people begin to cry when they first hear the Plants playing. Some tell me, "I know this song; I've heard it before." Hearing the Plants play this instrument is soothing and healing. I find their songs immediately put us in Heart coherence. What's more, most Plants enjoy playing—they like to hear themselves. I have witnessed that the Plants who sing become more vibrant and even retain their blooms for longer periods of time.

The Music of the Plants device is essentially a biofeedback machine that has been modified to read the electrical impulses from a Plant. There are two probes, a copper one which is inserted into the soil near the Plant's roots and an alligator clip that attaches to the Plant's leaf. These probes read the electrical impulses from the leaf and root. The device then translates the difference between these into musical notes.

What is particularly fascinating about this project is that it demonstrates that Plants can learn. The device can only read a limited number of possibilities, much less than what the Plant is capable of. Therefore, a Plant has to bring their electrical impulses into the range of the device and alter these so that the notes change.

Some Plants are more musical than others (and not all of them want to play). A Plant can start at any point on the continuum. At the very beginning of this continuum, a Plant does not play any notes; their impulses are out of range. Then they will play a note here or there. It is exciting to hear a Plant make a sound, but this is not a song. As the Plant continues to learn, they will start to play what I call scales. They start low and gradually play higher and higher notes before returning to the bottom of the scale again. They continue to repeat this. Then there is an intermediate step that some skip all together; it sounds like a Plant is playing a song, but if you listen closely, they are following the basic scales, starting low and going high, only with a little flourish added in. Eventually, if given time and if the Plant has the desire, they will begin to play their song.

This song is a reflection of the Plant's environment, including the emotional state of the humans. As a Plant becomes more proficient at the Music of the Plants instrument, they are more able to reflect their environment. I love to witness how a Plant adapts to the humans that come into their area. We have done experiments of having different people sit with a Plant and listening to the song change. But one of my most memorable experiences occurred with Pink Lady's Slipper. My friend and I spent a morning with Pink Lady's Slipper. I made an Essence while we listened to ki sing. It was my first time in this Forest; I didn't realize that we set up on top of a hill near a main trail. We listened to Pink Lady's Slipper sing for hours. At one point, ki suddenly stopped. About thirty seconds later, a couple came out of the Woods, rushing down the trail. After they were gone, ki started to sing again. This happened several times, though at times Pink Lady's Slipper continued to sing as people came down the trail and other times ki changed the song. It was clear that Pink Lady's Slipper was affected by the humans in the area and was able to sense them before we could.

Humans can play along with the singing Plants. This has also been an interesting experience to witness. My very first experience with this device was during a ceremony with Hawthorn held by Carole Guyett in Ireland. She connected a Hawthorn Tree to the device. At the time, I was with my Hawthorn friend when I heard the most angelic music. I apologized to my Tree; I needed to see where this music was coming from. I discovered that everyone else was converging on the same area and to our great surprise Hawthorn was creating the music. A friend began to play his flute. Then Carole's son joined in playing guitar and then Carole played her frame drum. I was entranced. If I closed my eyes, it sounded as if I was listening to a jam session between four musicians. They each took turns leading and they complemented each other well. I felt as if I was transported to another realm. Perhaps I was.

I am not a musician, therefore I do not know what is required to play with others. I thought that this experience was effortless. Since then, I have witnessed and heard from musicians that they struggle to play with the Plant. It seems that the Plant requires the human to listen and respond differently than what they are used to. The Plants are teaching them how to work co-creatively.

There are many amazing stories about this instrument. My absolute favorite experience with this device occurred in 2015. I was visiting Kauai'i, making Essences and teaching Plant communication. I brought the Music of the Plants device with me. My partner at the time was staying in a little community. People were curious about this device, so we decided to offer a concert. Since I was traveling, I did not have any singing Plants with me. I looked around the center and found a potted Plant who seemed to want to sing. I hooked ki up to the device and they began to play. (Some Plants are immediately proficient singers, while others can take months or longer to become performers.) I was grateful that ki was a good singer and was enjoying the music, when the gardener walked in. He immediately asked, "Where did you get that Plant!" I explained that I found ki outside and thought we could listen. This gardener had moved around for the past twenty years; he brought his beloved Begonia wherever he went. He stood in awe listening to the Plant play. Then he went over to Begonia and gently touched a leaf, ki played a note. He touched another leaf and ki played a different note. They continued to play like this, as if he was playing a Begonia piano. This extraordinary occurrence was obviously due to the extreme Love and reverence they shared for one another.

Dancing with Plants

When I share the Music of the Plants with groups, I ask them to stand up and dance for the Plants. Again, people become self-conscious. I encourage them to close their eyes and move their bodies. As they do, they hear the Plant responding to them. We have these remarkable bodies that allow us to move around. Plants appreciate when we dance with or for them. In many of my classes, we dance outside. This is not a time of worrying about steps or rhythm. There is no right or wrong way to move. We simply want to move because we can. As we move, we shift the energy around us, sending vibrations to the Plants. We can sense how our movement affects the Plants. We can also play around to see if there is a particular movement that a Plant likes. Maybe some want slow, rhythmic movements, or perhaps they like fast gestures. They might like it if we dance with them. As we dance with a Plant, we receive information. Dancing helps us to connect with our Plant ally.

Dancing with Plants is healing for us as well. It helps us to get in touch with our own bodies. So many of us are not fully embodied or tend toward dissociation. Dance brings our awareness to our body and encourages us to move in different ways. Dance gets our lymph flowing, enlivening us. And dance is downright joyful—a simple technique that benefits our health, gets us moving, helps us connect with our Plant, and adds more joy to the world. Let us all dance with Plants.

Making Apologies

The fields of my childhood have transformed from Tobacco and dairy farms to housing developments and shopping centers. Yes, we paved over (and continue to pave over) the beautiful, fertile soil of Lancaster County. We still have farms in Lancaster, just fewer. Some continue to be dairy farms, but driving around I mostly see Soybeans and field Corn (often GMO). Heart Springs Sanctuary is bordered by two such farms.

I used to cry and get angry when I saw another farm being transformed into buildings and asphalt. After observing my neighbors' farms and dealing with the enormous amount of runoff, I am no longer convinced that this is a horrible trade. I watch the water pour off of these farms, especially in the winter, just like ki does on asphalt. When your farm equipment is tractor trailers and you drive over this precious soil again and again and you remove all "competing" vegetation so that for half the year the field is barren soil, you create a compacted disaster.

I remember being a child and loving farms, believing that being a farmer meant working in partnership with Nature and learning from the Land. I remember, even as a young adult, visiting my grandfather's gardens and delighting in the colors and diversity, being in absolute awe of the generosity and abundance. This seemed like the closest one could be to the Divine. And for my minister grandfather, it was.

But as I look out at the surrounding farmland, I think, "This is not Nature." These are agro-industrial farms, an industry. The whole point is to override Nature because we are told that we can grow more and better food with technology and man's intelligence. But we can't and we need to accept this.

As I look out the windows, I can see one of the neighboring farms as well as part of the Sanctuary. They harvested the Soybeans last week; the farm is now flat and brown. I can't tell by looking, but I know that the Land is hard, almost like cement with debris poking up. This is in stark contrast to Heart Springs, which remains lush and green. There are many shapes and colors and heights. Bees, butterflies, other insects, and birds fly around the Sanctuary. Ki continues to glisten with the morning dew. When you step on the Land here, ki is soft and spongy. Last year, I hosted apprentices from California and Colorado. It was fire season when they left their homes and one of the first things that they noticed was the softness of the Land. Simply walking on this Land was healing. The irony is that most of what we have done at the Sanctuary is technically in violation of our local ordinances. According to these ordinances we are required to mow. Weeds are not supposed to be more than six inches high. Ragweed and Lamb's Quarter and other "weeds" tower over my head. And then there are the Trees who have sprouted and are well over ten feet tall.

One method increases biodiversity in both flora and fauna (aka, feeds life), increases carbon uptake, decreases water and soil runoff, helps to cool the Earth, and is illegal. Another method depletes soil, spreads poisonous chemicals, diminishes the capacity of soil to absorb carbon and water, increases water run-off, contributes to algal blooms in the Chesapeake, requires large amounts of fossil fuel thus contributing to air and noise pollution, and decreases biodiversity, yet is praised and subsidized.

As I drive by the fields of GMO Corn, I look at the wasted prayers. Who is praying to the Corn seeds as they are placed into the ground? Who is singing them alive? In the push for production and industrialization, we have forgotten our relationship with and responsibility to this Sacred Plant. Ki's adaptability has been abused to create new breeds that require poisons to grow and can be processed in a laboratory to create new foods, cleaning products, fuel, building supplies, plastics, and other products, but especially that pervasive, cheap sweetener, high fructose Corn syrup. Many of these new Corn based foods contribute to health issues, including diabetes, and are far removed from the nourishing foods ki provided that allowed the Indigenous to thrive before colonialism. Corn does not want to be a poison. Corn is the Great Mother who wants to nourish and help life to flourish.

It is time we apologized.

When I think of our relationships with Nature, I often think of humans as the addicts of the family. An addict will always be a part of the family, even if you try to cut them off. However, an addict is not able to fulfill their family role. They often aren't invited to gatherings, nor are they asked to help because they cannot be trusted. The family does not stop loving the addict. The other family members continue to pray and hope against all odds that the addict will remember who they are and return to the family. Unfortunately, the addict has a disease that keeps them hungry, and they will do anything to stop this hunger, even if just for a moment. The disease does not wipe out all of their memories; sometimes when they think of their family and who they have become, a great shame washes over them. They become paralyzed by this shame and the only way they know to erase shame is to numb themselves. An addict deflects responsibility, blaming others for their situation. Sometimes an addict experiences a reprieve and returns to the family for a while, but then they get pulled under again. Some addicts do not survive; they die never remembering the truth and beauty of who they are, never understanding that they are Sacred and loved so very much. And then there are the brave ones, who stare down their demons and return to the family. They may continue to struggle with the disease and amnesia, but every day they remain committed to honoring their Sacred role as part of this incredible family. As recovery programs have shown, some of the first steps to returning to the family are to admit our mistakes and to make amends. Sometimes this is overwhelming and can drive one back into their addiction, choosing amnesia. But for those who are able, making amends is freeing, it releases us from carrying the burdens, and helps us to repair our relationship. Fortunately, our relatives, especially Plants, have been hoping against hope that we will re-member. We have made many mistakes; whether they occurred at our hands or not does not matter—we allow them to continue. While making amends to Nature may feel like a daunting task, one apology begins our journey back into the family.

> *Great Mother,*
> *I am so, so sorry.*
> *I apologize for our forgetfulness and disrespect.*
> *I apologize for our manipulation and mutilation of*
>   *your genes.*
> *I apologize for the tons of poisons and chemical*
>   *fertilizers we have dumped on you.*
> *I apologize for the disappearance of your relatives, the*
>   *Insects and Birds, due to these poisons.*
> *I apologize for overprocessing you, turning you, your*
>   *Sacred self, into a poison, killing the humans with*
>   *disease.*
> *Great Mother, Grandmother, I apologize for separating*
>   *you from your other Plant friends so that we may*
>   *grow you in perfect rows.*
> *I apologize for the incessant push toward productivity.*

*I apologize for the silence, the missing prayers and
songs.
Great Mother Corn,
I apologize for the monstrous machines who have taken
over your planting, growth, and harvesting, who
cannot cradle you in their hands, staring in awe at
your beauty.
I apologize for the disregard of your precious Seed as
ki falls from tractors and trucks, scattering on the
roads, is left on the ground and piled high into
mountains of feed.
How we have forgotten the preciousness and celebration
of each and every Seed.
Grandmother Corn, I apologize for all this and so
much more.
But most of all, Great Mother, I apologize for the
murder, rape, and oppression of your People, the
Corn People, the Maize People.
This is where it all began.
We cannot hurt your People without hurting you and
we cannot hurt them without hurting ourselves, but
we broke the Sacred oath.
We have forgotten our connection to all of Life.
When we came to these beautiful, pristine Lands,
our disease of greed and insatiable hunger mistook our
relatives for commodities.
We sold and destroyed the very Beings who give us life.
Grandmother I am sorry, I am sorry.
I offer you my tears, may they quench your thirst and
water your Seeds.
I offer you my hands, may they be of service to you,
may they be instruments of Love repairing our
relationship.
I offer you my voice, may my songs nourish you, and*

*may I be an instrument for you, speaking up and
    calling us back into sanity and wholeness.
I ask you, Great Mother, Grandmother Corn, please
    show me how to make amends.
I give you my Heart, my Love, my awe, and my
    extreme gratitude.
Thank you for continuing to nourish us.
Thank you for holding Hope for us and staying when
    you could have disappeared.
Thank you for calling us back into relationship.
I hear you, I hear you.
We hear you.**

After expressing our apology, it is helpful to put energy behind our words. In this case with Corn, we can discover the varieties that the Indigenous grew in our area and plant these seeds, offering prayers and songs. We do not need to grow an entire field, but perhaps just a few Plants, even if they are in pots. We could donate to Indigenous organizations who focus on seed saving, seed sovereignty, and Indigenous seed rematriation. We could speak up about the harms of GMOs and industrial agriculture and encourage a shift toward farming in alignment with Nature such as regenerative agriculture. We could ask Corn how to best make amends. Whatever we do, may we be the brave ones who break the addiction, apologize, and return to the loving arms of our family.

Exercise: Engaging in Song and Dance with Your Plant Ally

It is time to connect with your Plant ally using sound. Gather any instruments that you have: rattles, drums, flutes, guitar, or your voice. If you

---

*While for years I have offered apologies in numerous ways to our more-than-human kin, after hearing V (formerly known as Eve Ensler) read her "Letter of Apology to Mother Earth" as part of her keynote talk, "The Alchemy of the Apology," at Bioneers in 2019, I was inspired to deepen my practice and give more of myself in my apologies. One of the results is this apology to Grandmother Corn.

have several options, you may want to do this process over several days, or you can bring them all out and have a jam session with your Plant.

⌀ Move into your Heart space and connect with your Plant ally.

⌀ Begin to play an instrument, hum, or sing.

⌀ Pay attention to how your Plant ally is responding as well as how your body is responding. Allow the music to bathe your Plant with Love. Are there any sounds that are naturally coming forward? Do you want to play softly, slowly, or fast? Does your Plant prefer one instrument over another? (You do not need to have multiple instruments; your voice is more than sufficient.)

⌀ There are tones that are connected to our chakras. They follow the C Major scale, as you can see in the following chart.

CHAKRA TONES

Chakra	Note	Sound
Root/1st	C / do	uh as in up
Sacral/2nd	D / re	ooo as in too
Solar Plexus/3rd	E / mi	oh as in so
Heart/4th	F / fa	aw as in saw
Throat/5th	G / so	i as in fly
First Eye/6th	A / la	ay as in play
Crown/7th	B / ti	eee as in tee

⌀ Try singing these tones with your Plant. Notice if one feels more harmonious to you or if your ally seems to respond more to a particular note. How does your body respond to these? You can then try other tones, sing a note or several and allow your Plant ally to interact with you. As you do this, pay attention to what is happening around you. Are birds joining in? What other sounds do you hear? Has the energy shifted?

⌀ As you sing, or perhaps on another day, begin to move your body. How does your Plant respond? Move in funny ways, with large steps and arm movements. While dancing, concentrate on your connection with your Plant. Let your movements be an honoring. Does your Plant want to dance with you? Do they enjoy the large movements or do they like fluid movements? How do you feel as you dance with your Plant? Let your body express your Heart.

🍂 Be sure to write down your experiences and any observations.

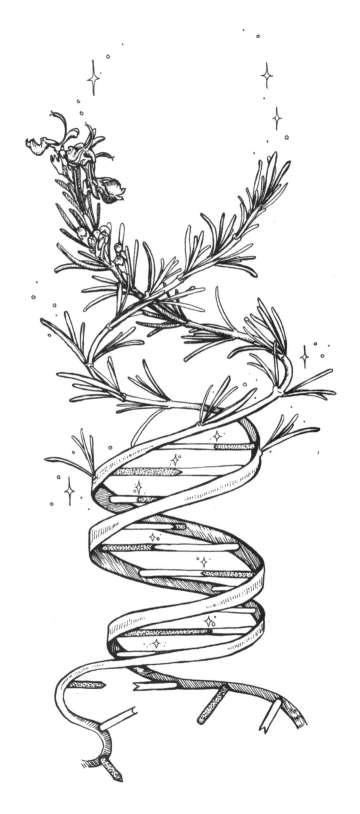

16
❧ Re-membering a New Way ❧
Rosemary

*W*hile we have many apologies and amends to make, Nature is the great forgiver. I am beyond humbled by the extreme generosity of her forgiveness. Nature is rooting for us. If we make a mistake or do not learn a lesson, we will be given another chance, sometimes it may take hundreds of chances until we learn. Nature will continue to forgive and support us along the way.

As I write, I have a dead Rosemary Plant on my desk. This may seem like a strange admission, but it's true. Just because I know how to communicate with Plants does not mean that I don't make mistakes or that I don't kill Plants. The truth is that I am a Rosemary killer. I admitted this publicly when I inherited this Rosemary from my grandmother. Ki was beautiful, in a sweet pot with a little Faerie figurine. I know my past experience and wanted help to keep this Plant healthy. Only one person responded with a suggestion (spray Rosemary with water several times a week). Everyone else admonished me and suggested that I change my language. Yes, I know words are powerful. I did not accept this nickname to set an intention, but as a warning. See, I have murdered over twenty Rosemary Plants with incredible efficiency. Some of them die within days of acquiring them or bringing them into my house. Each death hurts my Heart and leaves me feeling guilty at my inability to provide what they needed. Yet whenever I go to a Plant sale, I hear Rosemary begging me to bring ki home. I've tried to talk them out of it, but they insist, believing that this time would be different. For a brief moment, I, too, would be hopeful, only to have my friend die again. Despite my murders, Rosemary continues to forgive me and wants to be in relationship with me.

Power of Forgiveness

For many of us, forgiveness is an elusive concept, something we relegate to Saints or people more evolved than us. We were taught as children to forgive and forget, which just didn't feel right to us—after all, we were hurt. Were we supposed to ignore our pain or someone's hurtful actions? Sometimes it feels as if we hurt ourselves again when we forgive someone who has hurt us. The problem is that we were led to believe that forgiveness is for someone else, when in reality, we are the beneficiaries.

Remember, forgiveness is a positive Heart impulse. Whenever we engage in the energy of forgiveness, we flood our Heart, helping ki to soften, strengthen, and become coherent. When we choose to hold on to a resentment or injury, we deplete our energy (and immune system). Resentment prevents us from experiencing the full beauty of life. We replay the instance, experiencing the hurt and trauma again and again, getting locked into a re-traumatizing cycle. Meanwhile, the person who committed the act is going about their life, often oblivious of the hurt they caused us. Forgiveness is about you, not the person who hurt you. Doc Childre writes, "Forgiving releases you from the punishment of a self-made prison in which you're both the inmate and the jailer."[1] Forgiveness frees us from the pain of the past and enables us to more fully experience the present. Why do we want to continue to hurt and punish ourselves? When we forgive, we make our own health and well-being a priority.

Forgiveness is a difficult concept within a society that focuses on retribution. If you did something "wrong," you need to be punished. The problem is that punishment does not heal the wound for either involved and usually the person who committed this act did so out of previous pain and trauma. Maybe we need to revisit Ruby Sales and the question, "Where does it hurt?" I think the real question is, do we want retribution or do we want healing? When we remember that we are all connected, we see that retribution does not serve anyone. We want everyone to remember their innate Sacredness and heal. Retribution and punishment only create more pain, often compounding the problem. We see this clearly in our criminal system. Rarely do offenders receive the care and support that they need to heal and turn their lives around. Instead, we put them in a system which Daniel Goleman refers to as "a psychopath's paradise, where coolheaded cruelty wins the day."[2]

Often when the subject of forgiveness is mentioned, we begin to feel guilt and shame because we know that we *should* forgive, but we haven't; therefore, there is clearly something wrong with us. Forgiveness feels like an impossibility. In reality, forgiveness is as easy as breathing; we simply make it harder than we need to. Most likely you participate in many acts of forgiveness throughout your day, but they do not involve triggering events, so you don't even notice them. Perhaps you can notice that you are not walking around angry at everyone. (Or if you are, then we want to focus on self-Love and self-nourishment and perhaps even grief before trying to engage with forgiveness.)

We can look to the Plants as our forgiveness ambassadors. How many times have we ignored a Plant, cut one down, trampled on one, or harvested one without even noticing? Think about all the acts of destruction humans have inflicted on Plants, including the times we forced Plants into acts of violence such as Trees used for lynchings or branches for whipping people and animals. And yet the Plants continue to provide the life-giving gift of oxygen as well as food, medicines, and other materials needed for our survival. They continue to bathe us in Love and try to get our attention. I have yet to have a Plant treat me as unworthy or want to punish me. I have harmed them again and again; I have murdered numerous Rosemary Plants and they forgive me over and over. They may suggest ways in which I can apologize or how I can make a situation better, but they do not shame or punish me.

Several years ago, I was driving down the road when, out of the blue, I experienced an incredible moment of forgiveness. Prior to this, forgiveness seemed elusive to me. Even more surprising, I wasn't even trying to engage in forgiveness. My dad is a recovered alcoholic. He and my mom divorced when I was little. After many years of addiction, my dad successfully chose sobriety when I was twelve. I was always Daddy's little girl and in my young eyes my dad could do no wrong. Something switched when I went to college—I realized that it was my mother who was always there for me. For many years afterward my relationship with my dad was strained. I'm not sure if he was even aware of this, but I was. I was angry and resentful. At the time, I was living a few blocks from where he grew up. One day as I left my house, I drove down the road thinking about my dad. I was able to catch a glimpse of what his childhood was like. As wonderful as my grandparents were to me, I know that they were not great parents for my father. Their fundamental Christian beliefs greatly clashed with my dad's hippie Piscean ways. Without a doubt, they loved him; he was the golden, miracle child. But they did not understand him and they definitely did not know how to nurture his Soul. As they all grew older, their relationship became infinitely easier, but I don't know if they ever really knew their son.

As I thought about my dad's childhood, I suddenly realized that my dad loved me the best that he could. He may not have been able to meet me in the manner in which I wanted, but that did not mean that he didn't love me with his whole Being. Suddenly, all the anger and resentment left my body. My Heart felt enormous and light, my body radiated warmth. I was at peace. I realized that I completely forgave my dad. What's more, I was released from the burden of resentment. I never told him about this experience. I also never told him how angry I was with him. But almost immediately our relationship started to change. My dad no longer needed to be anyone other than who he was. One of the great gifts of my father is that he never expected me to be anything other than who I am. We were now free to simply enjoy one another, free of any resentments or judgments or burdens. I still, however, needed to address any habitual behavior patterns or beliefs I had created based on my experiences with my dad.

Before we can forgive, we need to acknowledge our wound and feel the emotions. I find it best to do this when I'm alone and in a quiet, safe place or with the Plants. Sometimes I walk the Labyrinth or go for a gentle walk in the Woods. Other times I need to voice my experience and feelings and receive reflection or a different perspective. I can do this with a therapist or good friend; in either case, I am discerning about who I process with as I do not want their own limiting beliefs to influence my experience. As much as it may (briefly) feel good to have someone validate our pain and criticize the "offending" party, ultimately this does not help our growth. Depending on the hurtful action and connection to previous traumas, this process can last anywhere from a split second to many years. The key is to process this fully, feeling all you need to feel without judgment about the length of time. The process takes as long as it needs to take, and it is possible that we may need to revisit the pain and emotions several times.

As part of this first step, we want to be curious. Has this offending action brought up any old traumas? Am I upset about something else? Is my level of emotion in proportion to what was said or done? What need(s) do I have? (I find the Needs Inventory on the website of the Center For Nonviolent Communication helpful with this.) We may also need to do something to help us restore: perhaps engage in self-Love, take a bath, receive a massage, go for a walk, spend time with a friend, dance—whatever helps you to feel more present and grounded.

Once we have processed our pain and are able to access our Heart space we are more able to experience compassion and understanding. We tend to think that this is the difficult part of forgiveness—we don't want to have compassion for someone's "bad" behavior. Based on what I have witnessed, we are actually struggling with processing our own feelings. People are naturally compassionate. It is their wounds and fear of being hurt that prevent their compassion flowing forth. Again, it is easier to experience compassion when we have focused on our pain and are in our Heart space.

To experience compassion, we again want to become curious. But before we do that, it is helpful to remember that we are all human, we have all hurt people, and we all make mistakes. We are still learning and healing. I also like to remember Don Miguel Ruiz's second agreement: "Don't take anything personally."[3] It is helpful to understand that a person's behavior or words are not a reflection of me, but of them, their story, and their pain. Most people carry around more pain than they are willing to acknowledge, even to themselves. I personally want everyone to embrace their gifts and beauty. I do not want them to be less than who they are, nor do I want them to suffer (although I accept that sometimes suffering is part of learning). When we can see that their actions are a reflection of their pain, it becomes easy to forgive. It is also helpful to remember that this is about understanding, and not about excusing bad behavior.

For this stage, we want to get curious about why our loved one acted the way that they did. Depending on the situation and our relationship with them, we can simply ask what was going on for them. Other times it is helpful to get to know a little about their story. What was their childhood like? What is their life like now? Are they experiencing any challenges? What needs do they have? Were they reacting toward us? Did we do something or do we represent something that triggered them? It can be helpful to remember their young child self. Again, this may be a brief process or it may take years to fully understand. It may be helpful to work with Black-Eyed Susan to look at the situation from a different perspective.

Sometimes it is helpful to do Soul contract work. Before being born into this life, members of our Soul family agreed to help us learn certain lessons just as we agreed to help them learn theirs. But of course, as part of the amnesia we forget all of this and sometimes what is supposed to be a learning experience becomes a trauma. Our foundational lessons are with our primary family members (parents, siblings, and children); therefore, we begin by exploring these Soul contracts. It can be tempting to focus on our Soul contracts with other relationships. However, if we do not discover and embrace the foundational lessons with our primary family, these lessons will continue to appear, so it is best to heal and address this at the source rather than potentially having to go through multiple relationships. There is a reason that we attract people with personalities similar to our parents and continue to repeat patterns.

When people first learn about Soul contracts, they generally want to renegotiate and change things, because they clearly did not agree to this. However, this is rarely what is needed. Usually, our Soul contract work helps us to get a better understanding of or a different perspective on our relationship and experiences. When we know the lessons that we wanted to learn and see how our loved one was helping with them, the house of cards we built on our perceived traumas comes tumbling down and our relationships shift.

During my divorce, I looked at my Soul contract with my ex-husband. As part of the lessons, he agreed to help me embrace my strength and stand up for myself. I was in awe. While I did not like the manner in which I learned this lesson, he definitely helped me learn it. Things shifted for me with this new understanding; I could see the Love in his actions. I still did not want to be married nor did I want to spend time with him, but on a Soul level I knew that we were good and I appreciated his assistance.

This process of understanding is not straightforward; we often move in and out of our pain and our compassion. When we have embraced our pain, taken care of our needs, and felt compassion and understanding for our loved one, then forgiveness naturally flows. We feel our Hearts opening, our bodies relaxing, and an overall release. We may even feel euphoric or blissful. Usually Love comes flooding forward. Once you feel this, you will want to continue to engage with forgiveness. Because again, *you* are benefiting from forgiving. You are free from that jail. You released the burdens and fed your Heart. You are more able to experience the beauty of life. Jonathan M. Goldman writes, "By my forgiving, I don't change what happened in the past. But I completely change my own future."[4] You have regained authority of your life and future.

Forgiveness feels incredible, and we do not stop here. A main stumbling block for many people is the perception of excusing the behavior, which can be how the forgetting part of "forgive and forget" is interpreted. But that is not how I understand forgetting. For me, forgetting is erasing the trauma from my body and possibly even my story line, not excusing abusive behavior. However, depending on the situation, I may need to set some boundaries with this person, perhaps even ending our relationship. I can continue to love them and forgive them, but I may need to do this from a distance for my own safety and self-Love. We do not need to be doormats or punching bags, continuing to allow ourselves to get hurt by people who are unable to meet us how we need them to. This is not about punishment or retaliation; it is about recovering trust and repairing the relationship. As part of this, we may need to accept the role that we played. Were we ignoring the needs of our loved one? Did we ignore signs? Are there traumas or patterns that we need to heal or shift? Remember, every moment of conflict is an opportunity to learn and heal, no matter how uncomfortable it is.

We need to remember to forgive ourselves as well, both for the pain we have caused others and for the pain we have experienced. Bessel van der Kolk says, ". . . the thing about being hurt is that when you feel hurt, you always hate yourself for getting hurt: I wasn't strong enough. I didn't resist enough. I didn't fight back. I didn't whatever. There's this deep sense of hating yourself for allowing whatever bad happened to you."[5] We need to understand that we did the best that we could at the time and forgive ourselves. When we release ourselves from this burden, we experience deep healing, dissolving the need to project this pain onto others and stopping a vicious cycle of wounding.

Balancing Intelligences

Throughout this book, I have stressed the importance of listening to the wisdom and intelligence of Nature, often while ignoring our own brains and egos. Human intelligence is a great gift. I am a firm believer in lifelong learning. The issue is that through our domestication, we have forgotten that we possess many different forms of intelligence, while also ignoring the possibility that our more-than-human relatives are intelligent—and in many ways. Therefore, it is important to shift out of brain-centered intellect when we begin our exploration into Plant communication. However, once we are comfortable experiencing these other forms of intelligence and moving into union with our Plant ally, we can incorporate our intellect into our experiences. By doing so, we create a future of balanced healthy relationships, where humans are part of the circle, one voice among many, co-creating the future together with all other Beings. Humans are capable of incredible ingenuity and creativity; I can only begin to imagine what a marvelous world we can create when we combine these with the extraordinary gifts and wisdom of our more-than-human kin. This is what gives me hope for our future.

In the Eastern Hemlock chapter, I shared the example of the time that we ignored the guidance of Nature and chose to follow our own human wisdom instead. The issue here wasn't that Marcus found another Tree he thought was a better option. The problem was that we didn't take this information back to the Nature Spirits or inform anyone about our intentions. From the perspective of the community of the Trees, I believe that the Hemlock Tree that the Nature Spirits had picked out was the best option. However, Marcus had a valid point that it would have been incredibly challenging to get to this Tree and to cut and remove ki, especially since ki would need to fall on our neighbor's Land. Had we shared this information with the Nature Spirits, we would have created a way forward together. That is what we are looking for—a future where humans work together *with* the other Beings of Nature.

Humans have different gifts and limitations than the other Beings of Nature. The Nature Spirits do not always understand these, so it is helpful for us to share our wisdom and limitations with them. When the Nature Spirits want me to make an Essence at three in the morning, sometimes I agree and other times I explain that I need a good night's sleep and then ask whether it is most important that this Essence be made now, or whether we can make the Essence at another time. Sometimes we are limited by financial resources, and we let them know our requirements. They can help us receive what is needed in many different ways.

Our amnesia and domestication have made us more of a burden than a blessing. Yet we are Nature. When we remember that our voice is neither more nor less valid than Blue Jay's or Sweet Gum's or the Susquehanna River's or that of another human, we are able to be in healthy relationship and to share our wisdom and perspective as necessary. We become an asset, adding to the beauty of Earth.

It is important that we continue to learn and study different ways of experiencing the world, be that by studying herbalism, homeopathy, biodynamic agriculture, astrology, painting, playing the cello, cooking, knitting, or whatever stirs your Heart. As we learn, we broaden our perspective. The wisdom of Nature is infinite, but often we need to have a context to understand the information that we receive. I understood the image of the hügelkultur bed for the Blueberries because I was already aware of this form of gardening, which enabled me to ask more questions about the specific components.

I asked for help with Rosemary from my human friends because so far I have not found a way to keep ki alive. I believe it is possible; I know that it is—many people grow Rosemary. I have done research, I have communicated with Rosemary, I have experimented, and I haven't found the solution. It feels as if there is a block somewhere, something that I am not getting or that I need to learn. Therefore I reached out, hoping that someone who grows Rosemary could give me advice that they have found to be successful. As sad as I am that this sweet Plant died, I know that if I am meant to learn this lesson, I will. For now, though, I keep this Rosemary here to honor and mourn. I continue to bathe ki in Love, knowing that Rosemary Plant Spirit can sense this.

Karma

The Hindu concept of karma has been adopted into the Western world to signify reward or punishment for actions. This is connected to our belief of good and evil. Seeing karma in this manner feeds our belief in retribution: if you are a good person, you will receive your just rewards (in this life or the afterlife) and if you are a bad person, you will be punished. If life is not going well for you, then you are clearly being punished. And if you are rich, wealthy, and life is easy, then you are simply being rewarded, and you should accept your rewards without any concern about others. But anyone who has taken the effort to connect with people outside of their comfort zone can tell you that this is bullshit. Your financial status and the ease in which you move through life has very little to do with whether you are "good" or "bad."

I am neither Hindu nor a yogini; however, my experience with what I believe to be karma is very different from the Western worldview. Karma is not a system of reward and punishment. Karma is simply there to help us learn our lessons, heal, and evolve. If we do not learn a lesson in this life, we will have an opportunity to learn it again in the next. In the meantime, lessons will continue to arise. If a pattern continues to repeat itself (you date people who end up being jerks, or you repeatedly get fired, or every time you decide to do something for yourself, something occurs that blocks this experience), pay attention; either there is a lesson that needs to be learned or something needs to be healed. Sometimes this is connected to a past life, but not always. The Plants can help us to heal and understand our lessons. Mostly, they want us to know that we are not being punished; our lessons are for our own growth. We live in the Universe of Perpetual Second Chances. If we mess up or do not learn a lesson the first time, we'll be given another chance—this is karma. When we do learn a lesson, I imagine that a little celebration occurs in the Spirit realm: "Yay! They're getting it! Look at them growing and evolving!"

Ancestors

Rosemary is well known as a Plant for remembrance—as in, ki enhances our memory. Rosemary also helps us to connect and honor our Ancestors. As we saw with Black-Eyed Susan, our Ancestors can affect us even without our awareness through inherited beliefs and traumas. They are also an enormous resource for support and guidance. We have lost much ancestral wisdom, especially in the United States. This is in part due to people losing (consciously or unconsciously) connection with their families and Ancestors when they immigrated. Then there is the forced disconnection caused by slavery and the systemic oppression and genocide of Native Americans.

Our Ancestors helped to form and give meaning to our life. If we do not know them or our family stories and traditions, we cannot fully know ourselves. The colonizers knew this and consciously made decisions (and laws) to break the ancestral ties and obliterate the ancestral wisdom of both Native Americans and Black people. It is easier to control and manipulate orphans who do not know the truth of who they are. Rosemary helps us to acknowledge and remember our Ancestors whether we know them or not, and can help us to regain our ancestral wisdom. Wisdom can never be truly lost, only temporarily forgotten.

Our family Trees are not always neat and tidy. There can be multiple forks due to divorce, death, adoption, or other reasons. Rosemary can help us to heal and honor any of these ancestral lineages. Our Ancestors do not need to be blood relatives. Nor do we need to know who they are. These limitations do not exist in the other world.

There are many ways to honor and reconnect with our Ancestors. We can learn about our heritage, make and eat ancestral food, visit ancestral Lands, go on a journey to meet them or spend time with them, create an altar with photos of them or items that are connected to them, give offerings, light candles for them, share family stories or songs, celebrate family traditions or learn the traditions of your heritage, or plant Trees or Plants that are connected to them. There is no shortage of ways to connect; do what feels powerful and meaningful to you. One way of strengthening your relationship with your Ancestors is to ask for their assistance. They love us and want to help us to evolve and thrive. Even if we had a difficult relationship with them when they were alive, once they are in the Soul world, all is well; they are in the place of infinite Love. We can connect with our Ancestors at any time, but the veil between our world and the ancestral or spiritual world becomes thin near the end of October and the beginning of November. This is the time of year when it becomes easier to connect with them. You may want to pay attention to your dreams during this time or hold a special ceremony to honor them.

As we discover our Ancestors, we may find ourselves drawn to certain lines or stories while wanting to ignore other aspects of our family's past. We all have oppressors and the oppressed in our ancestry; both need healing. Our work is focused on healing and releasing the burdens, without judgment. We need to face the pain as well as the harm done and appreciate the joys and gifts. Ignoring them or changing the narrative does not free us from the burdens. Pam Montgomery writes, ". . . until we lay down the ancestral burden and refuse to carry it forward anymore, there can never be peace on this planet. Until we heal our ancestral line we will always be tormented by the longing of our ancestors and imprisoned by their grief. When they heal we can stand on their proud backs, giving our children courage to be happy descendants."[6] Engaging in ancestral healing benefits all of our relatives, our Ancestors, ourselves, and our descendants. Pam refers to this work as "healing the past to affect the future."[7] As we remember our Ancestors and release their burdens, we enable one another to focus more on our evolution and communal future.

There is much in this world that needs to be healed; the traumas continue to be passed down through generations. We can also heal the traumas and burdens of the Ancestors of the Land where we live. In my case, this would be the Susquehannocks. I find this work to be a little different than healing my ancestral lineage. Generally, I ask how to make amends and work with the Land. We can honor these Ancestors by learning about the Plants they grew or their cosmology. We can give them offerings, journey with them, or hold ceremonies to honor them. In my experience, they often simply want to be remembered and are delighted to guide our work with the Land.

Ancestral honoring and healing bring us back into the circle of our more-than-human family. If we follow our lineage back far enough, we meet our more-than-human Ancestors. As Michael Soulé writes, ". . . there is now no question that all life on earth evolved from a common ancestor. The genetic material and the codes embedded within it reveal that every living kind of plant and animal owes its existence to a single-celled ancestor that evolved some three and a half billion years ago. All species are *kin*."[8] We cannot escape our ancestry, they are part of our bodies. When I'm struggling, sometimes I like to pause and think back through the lineages down to the cyanobacteria and the primordial stew that have enabled my life at this moment in time. My mind cannot really grasp it, but there is a sense in my body of the enormity of choices, actions, challenges, and connections that have led to this moment. Just thinking about all the lives who enabled our existence is humbling. My response is of awe and gratitude, which turns into responsibility, both to my Ancestors and to the future generations. We owe them so much.

Re-membering Our Wholeness

As we heal and evolve, we discover that we have the great gift and responsibility of creating ourselves and our lives. We can choose the qualities we incorporate into our life and body as well as the energies we want to resonate with. Rosemary helps to shift our internal environment to be in alignment with our Essence or Truth. Ki literally helps us to re-member, to put ourselves back together into our wholeness. Rosemary enables us to override our traumas and limiting beliefs and remember the beautiful, perfectly imperfect Soul we began this life with adding in the lessons and growth we've experienced, so that each cell of our body knows the Truth: we are Love(d) and we are connected to all.

Rosemary Plant Spirit takes the threads of separation and reweaves them into our family tapestry, reminding us that we are an intricate part of this exquisite fabric we call Nature. As ki weaves, Rosemary heals the separation of our own body, bringing into harmony our Heart, Soul, and Spirit, so that we may live the life of our Soul's yearning. We remember the gifts and guidance that surround us. We remember our role as co-creators. We remember our inner child. We remember our Wise One within. We remember our Heart's desire. We remember how to live in harmony with all life. We remember that we are Sacred Divine Beings. As we remember, we re-member, bringing to life those aspects of ourselves we thought were gone or unattainable. We remember all that we are and all that we can be. As we remember, we help others to re-member themselves. We hold the image of their Sacred selves, calling them back to themselves. The more who remember, the more we are able to collectively re-member. Our more-than-human relatives sense this; they sense our awakening, our re-membering, and they rejoice. They are grateful to welcome us back into the family. Rosemary guides us in re-membering our future. Together, we thrive.

Exercise: Co-creating Your Plant Ally's Story

You have experienced different methods for communicating with your Plant ally. Now is the time to co-create ki's story. In the herb world, we call these Plant monographs.

🖋 As you review your notes and reflections from previous exercises, look for repeated messages or patterns. Is there a theme throughout your experiences? Was there a moment that was particularly powerful or explicit?

● Compile the threads of information you've received. What are the healing gifts of your Plant? What have you learned by spending time with your Plant ally? What questions do you still have? How are you to work with this Plant? What does the Plant want from you?

● As you begin to put together your Plant ally's story, you may want to reference what others have written about your ally. Remember that each Plant meets you where you are and we could never compile all of the gifts and messages that a Plant provides. Still, it is helpful to read what others have said. Sometimes this is validating and other times it can help make sense of an experience or message. There are many wonderful resources for discovering more about Plants. Some of my favorites are:

> The Book of Herbal Wisdom by Matthew Wood
> The Energetics of Western Herbs by Peter Holmes
> Flower Power by Anne McIntyre
> Native American Medicinal Plants by Daniel E. Moerman
> Plants Have So Much to Give Us, All We Have to Do Is Ask by Mary Siisip Geniusz
> Stars of the Meadow by David Dalton
> Working the Roots by Michele E. Lee

● This is the time to bring discernment into your experience with the Plant. Now that you have had many experiences, you have a greater context for understanding. There may be some messages or experiences that you are uncertain about, that perhaps were influenced by something going on in your life (which does not necessarily negate their accuracy). For these, I simply leave a question mark. As I continue to communicate with the Plant, I may find more information about these situations.

● When you feel you have compiled and organized the information received from your Plant ally, you may want to share this with others. It is helpful to have others hear our experience. Sometimes they can help us make sense of it and other times they validate what we received.

● Remember that this is only the beginning. You can continue to learn from and communicate with your Plant ally for years and years. This is a lifelong relationship. Your Plant ally will be there for you whenever you need them.

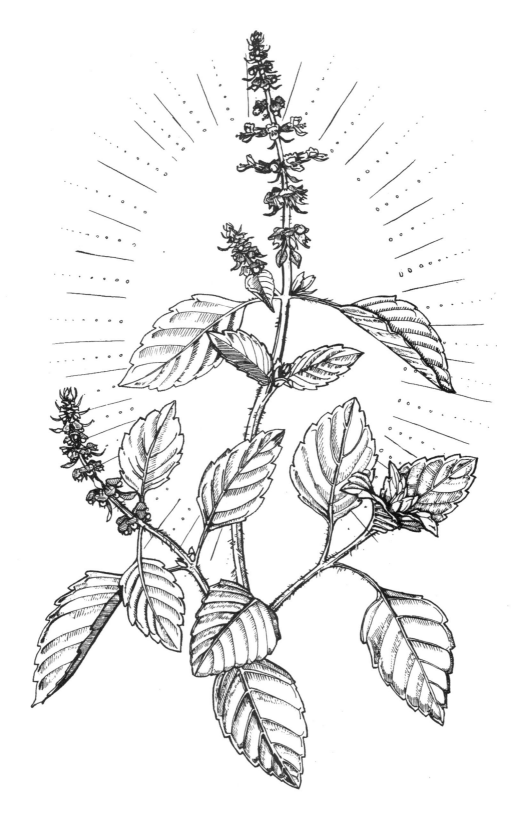

17
⤳ Becoming Sacred Humans ⤳
Tulsi

One whiff of Tulsi, also known as Holy Basil, Sacred Basil, and Tulasi, and my Heart immediately opens while my body relaxes. *Tulsi* is a Sanskrit word meaning "the incomparable One." As ki's common name suggests, Tulsi is considered a Sacred Plant, revered in both Hinduism and Christianity. Yash Rai writes, "The Hindu scriptures enjoin us to look upon Tulsi not as a mere plant, but as the divine representative of the God Vishnu or of Lord Krishna."[1] And later Rai states, ". . . Tulsi has been given the apellation [*sic*] of 'Mother of the Universe'."[2] Anyone who has spent time with Tulsi understands this reverence, for ki seems to transport you to a place of peace, opening your Heart, and surrounding you with Love.

One year during the HEARTransformation Apprenticeship, we experienced a Tulsi Plant diet. It was a beautiful, sunny, warm, autumn day as we sat by Tulsi in the garden and sipped and nibbled on different preparations of ki's medicine. After the second or third preparation, I remember looking at my students and beaming with Love for them; I saw their perfection and was incredibly honored to share this time with them. After maybe one or two more preparations, I didn't want to leave the moment. I experienced a deep calm and the feeling of "this is it," as if all of life was meant to arrive at that moment, the moment of complete peace and complete Love. I could feel the deep connection with all, the Oneness of life. As the guide, I knew that I needed to lead us on, and yet I wanted to stay in the bliss of Tulsi.

It is not surprising to me that this Sacred Plant from India has become popular. We are able to find Tulsi in almost any grocery store. Ki is an important Plant for our times. Tulsi reminds us of our connection and opens our Hearts, helping them to connect to the Holy Heart, the place of Oneness. I have yet to meet someone who has not fallen under Tulsi's spell if given the chance. When I first met my dear friend Lisa Brinton, she did not like Tulsi; the scent made her sick. I was astonished and encouraged her to get to know the Plant. Now Lisa is one of the biggest advocates for Tulsi, sharing ki in ceremonies with her students.

Slower Than Slow

Humanity is moving at warp speed. We are addicted to the busy-ness of life. We have become adrenaline and cortisol junkies. Stress, caffeine, and sugar fuel us. This speed, this frenzy is part of the capitalism paradigm of production and competition. We always need to do more, there's very little time. As a double Aries, I get a glimpse of an idea and I'm flying ahead while everyone else is just beginning to wonder what is going on. But this speed is not in alignment with Nature. Don't get me wrong, Nature can make things occur instantaneously. But there isn't the frenzy. In general, Nature holds the long view.

Tulsi teaches me to slow down. We have a dance. I slow to what I consider an excruciatingly slow pace and ki says, "Slower." Tulsi's guidance is "Slower than slow." While I can get frustrated with this, after all there's much to do, there are moments when I understand the wisdom, as in the experience I described with my students. When we slow down, we are more able to appreciate the gifts of life. We can tap into the Love that surrounds us. Busy causes us to focus on the problems and what needs to be done. Slow asks us to look around and truly see the world. Often problems melt away as we witness the perfection of that moment. As I slow, Tulsi tells me, "Magic is in the in-between spaces." When we move too fast, when we are always busy, we miss the magic. Tulsi reminds us that we are human *Be*ings. It is important that we slow down and be.

Sometimes the best thing that we can do to create change in this world is to simply be. When we allow ourselves to be in this place of connection and appreciation, we realign the energies of our bodies. We remember who we are. This shift ripples out. We create the world from a place of peace, Love, and connection by simply slowing and being. We carry this energy with us as we go back to our activities. I remind myself that I am not only more productive, but also more effective and efficient when I take the time to slow down, be, and connect with my more-than-human kin. This makes sense, since we know that when we slow down and connect, we move into our Heart space and when we experience Heart coherence, we become more solution-focused, creative, and gain a broader perspective.

Tulsi is an adaptogen, meaning ki helps us to be more resilient during moments of stress. Whether we take the time to "be" or not, Tulsi helps us to remain healthy and happy in an increasingly stressful world. We know that happiness feeds our immune system. It appears that we could all use a little extra boost, both of immune support and happiness.

Soul Healing

Tulsi is a foundational Plant in Plant Spirit Healing. We work with ki whenever we engage in Soul healing such as karmic healing, Soul contracts, and Soul retrievals (bringing back parts of ourselves that we have lost along the way, often due to trauma). I have worked with Tulsi in countless sessions for my clients. It is always an honor when I am able to work with ki. Tulsi Plant Spirit is quite sweet, and ki is a fierce protector when needed.

Some of us are aware of previous lives; we may have memories or simply a sense of gnowing. Sometimes the lessons from those lives bleed into our present life. These can present themselves through illnesses, injuries, or wounds, especially if they occur on the right side of our body. We may also have made pacts or developed a belief in a previous life that impacts this one. For example, if our Heart was badly broken or we were betrayed, we may have said that we would never love again. In our present life, we have great difficulty with romantic relationships. We would like to experience Love, but whenever we are heading that way, something happens to end it. Another frequent belief or pact that I've witnessed with my clients is that they did something in a previous life that resulted in a person getting sick or the destruction of something, which they believed to be bad. They blamed themselves for this and then in this lifetime they are not able to trust their abilities or do not want to engage in their Soul Path. Tulsi helps them to understand why something occurred or what their lesson was, which helps to release them from this belief or pact, bringing healing. This is what we call karmic healing, when we can heal the energetic imprints from our other lives. Again, something that we determined to be bad when looked at in a different way may end up being exactly what was needed at the time. Karmic healing is incredibly freeing and empowering, allowing us to no longer be held hostage by our past lives or deeds. Sometimes we need to make amends, but often we discover that we have been tormenting ourselves for no reason.

If we want to be conscious adults, embracing who we are meant to be, we need Soul healing. In this amnesiac world, it is next to impossible to grow up without experiencing trauma or losing parts of ourselves. Robert Bly writes about "the long bag we drag behind us." This bag is filled with the parts of ourselves that our parents didn't like or our teachers or our peers or our partners until the bag becomes quite full and long. He writes, "We spend our life until we're twenty deciding what parts of ourself to put into the bag, and we spend the rest of our lives trying to get them out again. Sometimes retrieving them feels impossible, as if the bag were sealed."[3] If we fill this bag with enough parts of ourselves, we begin to feel diminished. Our light is dim, sometimes to the point where we do not have the will to carry on. This diminished light makes us easy targets for disease and negative energies.

Everyone benefits from doing Soul work, but if we are experiencing this level of depletion, Soul work is absolutely necessary. Through Soul retrievals, Tulsi helps us to remove these parts from the long bag, bringing us into alignment with wholeness. As we welcome our parts back, often memories return along with more vital energy. We have a greater sense of self. It is a special moment when a client is ready to have their Soul parts returned; how wonderful to witness a person experiencing this deep healing. Pam Montgomery writes, "Soul retrieval is integral to Plant Spirit Healing because the entire point of the practice is to help a person become more fully who they are, living according to their true nature and walking the path they came to walk this time around."[4]

Occasionally Tulsi helps us bring back a Soul part from a previous life. This is significant, as we are experiencing both karmic healing and a Soul retrieval, and we have been missing this part and their gifts for our entire lives. Perhaps my most profound healing experience was a retrieval of a Soul part from a past life. In this previous life, I experienced Sacred Love, which was ecstatic and extraordinary. Unfortunately, my role in my community did not allow for falling in Love, so I had broken the rules. I was unwilling and unable to give up this Love, and ended up losing both my community and my Love. I was devastated and chose to kill myself. Because I did not finish my lifetime, I did not complete my lesson. In my present life, I had a confusion between Sacred sex and Sacred Love. I was not able to experience Sacred Love because this aspect of myself was missing. My relationship with Marcus began shortly after my Soul part returned. I am now able to experience a level of Love and intimacy I could never have imagined before. I will forever be grateful to Tulsi.

These are only part of Tulsi's healing gifts. If you are feeling a deep Soul yearning or Soul level exhaustion or you simply know that something is happening on a Soul level, ask Tulsi for guidance. Ki is willing to help us. There is no need to suffer alone. Ultimately, Tulsi enables us to embrace our wholeness by re-membering who we are. The more healing we experience and the more we align with our Soul Path, the happier we become. Our relationships, romantic and not, are healthier and more fulfilling. We naturally attract people who support our becoming, our blossoming, and life in general becomes easier and more enjoyable. It doesn't mean that there aren't difficulties or challenges, but overall, we are able to truly love life. At least, this has been my experience since choosing to follow my Soul Path. I am continually in awe and often in tears when I think about the absolutely amazing people who have come into my life since I said "Yes!" to Yarrow. Their friendship and support have helped me through some arduous times and have led to beautiful adventures. I know that my personal work continues. As I say to my clients, I'm still alive, which means there is still healing work to do. And I'm excited to continue on this journey of Becoming and evolving with the Plants.

From my work with the Plants, especially Tulsi, I know that they are encouraging us to move into alignment with our inner divinity, truly becoming Sacred Humans. As a Sacred Human, we live in a way that honors the innate Sacredness of all Beings, including ourselves. This is who we are being asked to be, this is who we are. Or at least this is who we came to this world to be (without the amnesia). Through their guidance and healing work, the Plants help us to remember. The old story that we are sinners or less-than or unworthy is not true. No matter what your inner critic may say or what others have told you, you are a Divine Being. You may have made mistakes, possibly even big ones that have hurt other people, but this doesn't change the truth of who you are. No matter what you do or don't do, you cannot change who you are at the very Essence of your Being. As Jerry Tello says, "You are sacred, you are a blessing, just the way you are."[5] We need to believe this down into our very DNA, soaking our cells in our innate Sacredness. The Plants are calling, our other relatives are waiting, our future generations are depending on us to re-member our wholeness and become Sacred Humans.

Ceremony

When we engage in ceremony, we consciously engage with the Unseen world, uniting the physical and spiritual worlds. Ceremony feeds the Unseen and brings meaning to our lives. A portal is opened through ceremony, which facilitates communication and allows us to receive guidance or healing or share our intentions for this world. Indigenous cultures recognize the importance of ceremony, not only for living in alignment with Nature but also for nurturing the growth and evolution of their people.

For many living in Western cultures, ceremony seems like a foreign concept beyond our understanding and ability. And yet even in our modern culture, we have ceremonies, such as weddings or family traditions around holidays. Ceremonies can be large elaborate events where every detail is consciously chosen, or they can consist of simply making a cup of tea or lighting a candle. Ideally, we engage in ceremony every day. What sets ceremony apart from our everyday actions is our intention. We take even a brief moment to recognize the alchemy that occurs as we pour boiling water over dried Plants. We give thanks for both the water and the Plants and all the Beings who helped to grow them. We fill this tea with our intentions, prayers for the Earth, or Love. We may offer some to the Earth or pour ki in a tiny bowl for Faeries. As we drink the tea, we again express gratitude for ki's healing and open ourselves to receiving the blessings of this wonderful gift, taking a moment to commune with the Plant Beings.

Sacred Humans understand that every act, every word, every thought is an opportunity to feed the Unseen and create a world of beauty. When we walk barefoot on Earth, we receive the healing gifts of the Plants through the pores of our feet. With each step, we can infuse the Land with our Love and prayers. How different does this feel from rushing and not paying attention to our interaction with the Land below us? Even concrete and asphalt can receive our Love and radiate this throughout the city. Spirit loves beauty. As we dress in the morning, we can consciously adorn ourselves to bring beauty into the world, or choose clothes or jewelry that provide protection or enliven us. Every act, every word, every thought becomes a conscious act helping us to remain in Integrity, deepening our connection with Nature, feeding Spirit and our own Soul. Ceremony becomes a way of life.

Participating in a group ceremony can be particularly transformative and powerful, for you are combining the intentions of all involved often to create a change. The Organization of Nature Evolutionaries (O.N.E.) holds biannual Earth ceremonies. During these ceremonies, we ask people to participate around the world, focusing on a particular intention, perhaps gratitude for Trees or water. We provide a suggested format, but what is most important is that there is a large group of people focusing together, magnifying our prayers and intentions.

In large ceremonies, it is helpful to follow a particular format, which usually includes setting Sacred space before beginning. Following a format or structure time after time facilitates the ceremonial process. It is like walking on a trail through the Woods as compared to forging a new path every time. That being said, it is still recommended that we stay open to spontaneity and the energies that arise, for this is where the magic occurs. There really is no limit as to what encompasses a ceremony. We tend to think of ceremonies as somber affairs; they can just as easily be riotous, joyful celebrations filled with laughter and playfulness.

For eons, humanity has engaged in ceremony with Plants. We do this to honor them and show our gratitude, to receive healing for ourselves or others, or to help us visualize and receive guidance. Having a ceremony with your Plant ally is another opportunity for deepening your connection.

One of the great sadnesses of colonialism and the amnesia of separation is that many of us have lost the ceremonies of our Ancestors, including the initiations that marked life's thresholds. We lost those moments that helped us to understand who we are and that gave meaning to life. Still, the Earth remembers these ceremonies. We can ask our more-than-human kin to help us remember. Or perhaps, it is time to create new ceremonies that support us in our evolution.

Sacred Plant Initiations

Once again, the Plants offer us a solution: they will initiate us. In ceremonies called Sacred Plant Initiations, Plants guide us through our evolution, bring us back into the family, and help us to become Sacred Humans. Engaging in Sacred Plant Initiations opens us to a deeper understanding of and greater intimacy with our Plant ally.

Cultures around the world engage in Plant Initiations (sometimes referred to as Plant dieting or dietas) often with psychotropic Plants such as Ayahuasca, San Pedro, or Peyote. In her book, *Sacred Plant Initiations,* Carole Guyett shares how we can participate in similar ceremonies with the common (non-psychoactive) Plants who grow all around us. Carole writes, "Ceremonial plant dieting is a traditional method of honoring the plant world. The ceremonial process offers a unique way to connect deeply with all aspects of a plant, opening gateways to spiritual realms and facilitating powerful transformation at physical, emotional, mental, and spiritual levels."[6]

I have participated in and facilitated numerous Sacred Plant Initiations (the first initiation that I led was with Tulsi). Many of the messages that I shared in this book came forward during these ceremonies. The initiation usually occurs over two or three days. During this time, we fast (which is optional) and ingest a special elixir that is made with the Plant who is initiating us. We engage in ceremony the entire time, continually deepening our connection with the Plant. The contents of the elixir as well as the format for the initiation are guided by the Plant.

My experiences with Sacred Plant Initiations have been life changing. Sometimes the effects are immediate and other times it takes years for the pieces to fall into place. Regardless, spending a weekend in deep ceremony with Plants and wonderful humans nourishes my Heart and Soul. I leave these weekends feeling more alive and aligned and hopeful for our future. I engage with Plants and Plant Spirits every day; however, I experience a different connection during Sacred Plant Initiations. This connection carries onward. Carole shares, "Being initiated by a plant offers the possibility of merging with its consciousness. Thus, we can experience the connectedness of all life and thereby access Oneness through the plant world."[7] The initiation process continues long after the weekend is over.

While I absolutely love Sacred Plant Initiations and I am incredibly grateful to Carole for sharing these with the world, I am mindful about when I participate in one. This is not something that I do simply for the sake of doing or because I want an intense experience. I need to feel called by the Plant to deepen my relationship. I also need time in between the ceremonies to integrate my experiences and continue my relationship with the Plant (my Initiator).

Facilitating a Sacred Plant Initiation is an incredible gift, allowing me to experience the wonders of co-creative partnership. Again, I wait until a Plant steps forward and asks to be in ceremony. The Plant guides every step. Sometimes the preparation of the different components can take years to complete. I continue to be humbled and in awe of their generosity, forgiveness, and wisdom. Sometimes, I do not understand why they want something to occur a certain way or the language that they use, but inevitably it is exactly what someone needed. While the preparation is wonderful, the true magic occurs when the participants arrive. It is an enormous honor to witness the healing, re-membering, and changes that occur as humans move into intimacy with Plants. These weekends give me a brief glimpse into our potential future and I am filled with Love and admiration.

Becoming Alchemists

Mention alchemy and people think about the alchemists who were obsessed with turning lead into gold. But alchemy is much more than this. In simplest terms, alchemy is transformation. When we only consider alchemy as the pursuit of creating gold, it can seem like a ridiculous or failed ancient pursuit. This would be a mistake, for we experience alchemy every day. One could even argue that alchemy is the foundation of life.

Let's pause for a moment and contemplate the many transformations occurring. A Tree's leaves absorb sunlight and carbon dioxide to create nourishment for the Tree and, in the process, release oxygen for us to breathe. We take a deep breath and feel the gift of the Plants helping to calm our bodies, bringing us into present awareness. Sitting next to me is a cup of Tulsi tea, which was created by pouring boiling water over dried Tulsi leaves. I drink this warm concoction, breathing in ki's scent as I sip, and feel my Heart open. If I allow myself to pause and savor the tea and the scent, I can be transported back to the moment of bliss in the garden with my students. All of these are alchemy; transformation has occurred.

Transformation is an inevitable part of life. We can embrace ki's gifts and capabilities to facilitate our re-membering.

The goal of the ancient alchemists was to transform the dross into the pure. Some were corrupted by greed and confused these terms with material substances and financial wealth. They thought that money, particularly an unlimited source of money, could turn one into a God. Tulsi reminds us that the center of all—the purest substance—is Love. We become Divine Beings or Sacred Humans by aligning with Love.

One of the main components of alchemy is the container. The purer the container, the purer the creation. For the alchemy of life, our container is our energetic body. Tulsi helps us to release the dross, those aspects or experiences that prevent us from aligning with Love. These may be our traumas, beliefs, or fears. Tulsi gently helps us remember our Truth, our wholeness. The more we work with Tulsi, the more ki helps us to choose Love in all our actions. The more we choose Love, the purer our container becomes.

Choosing Love can be challenging for our culture does not support this path. It is easier to react with anger, othering, or fear. But these will not create a more loving world, these will not help us to become Sacred Humans, nor to thrive. When you begin to choose Love, you can feel the transformation in your body. For example, in an argument, you know that you could cut someone with your words, and you can feel the pull to follow that well-worn path. But you have made an agreement to Love; you know that hurting another person does not lead to Love. Instead of snapping back, you choose vulnerability, to express your needs and wonder about the other person's needs or wounds. You choose curiosity and connection, which elicits a bodily sensation. Often at first, there is discomfort because it is a new course. Ultimately, there is an uplifting, a ping and, frequently, there is a sweet surprise as the alchemy of Love transports you into a different experience. Another world opens. When we choose Love, we flow with the universe. This is the lesson of Tulsi.

When we get distracted or slip, falling back into old routines, Tulsi helps us return to our Hearts and realign with Love. Tulsi encourages us to embrace our innate alchemist, reminding us of our capabilities as Sacred Humans. As we become vessels of Love, we transform the world around us. We help others to align with their Truth. We help them to see the Sacred Beings that they are. Love is contagious.

Tulsi is the great mediator between Heaven and Earth, reminding us that they are one and the same. There is no separation. We can create Heaven on Earth; we can return to the Garden. The path is Love, and our Hearts know the way. Our Plant allies can help us remember whenever we are lost.

Exercise: Having a Ceremony with Your Plant Ally

Your relationship with your Plant ally is just beginning. This is a lifelong relationship, and it waxes and wanes; you may find that there are time periods where you want to connect with your Plant ally daily and then months or even years may go by without any interaction. As with all relationships, it is important to feed your connection with your Plant ally.

- For your final exercise, you are invited to engage in a ceremony with your Plant. This can be as simple or elaborate as you and your Plant would like. You could have a cup of tea with ki or engage in a three-day Sacred Plant Initiation or have a dance party or create a costume to embody your Plant or make a pact to honor ki with an action. There is no limit.

- Ask your Plant how ki would like to engage with you. Then plan the ceremony. If it feels right, invite your friends. We all benefit from engaging in ceremonies.

- To begin your ceremony, smudge or clear yourself and the space, then set Sacred space.
- Conduct your chosen ceremony.
- When finished, be sure to share your gratitude and reciprocity with your Plant friend and all the Guides who joined you. Close the circle.
- Add your experiences and observations to your Plant ally's story.

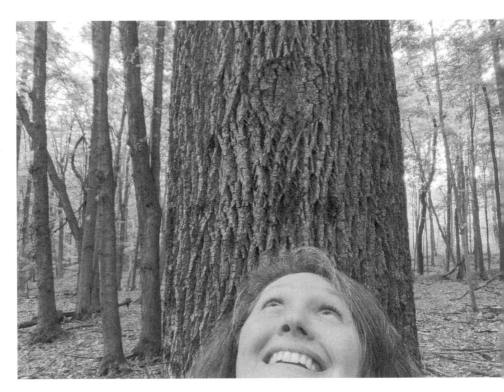

Author with her beloved Ash.

❧ Creating a New Story ❧

*W*hile this is the conclusion of this book, it is only the beginning—the beginning of your relationship with your Plant ally, your journey with Plant communication, and our re-membering. Throughout this book, I have shared repeatedly that when there is a need, a Plant will appear. Even my long-time students and clients ask me what they should do when they need support and I respond, "Ask for a Plant." When a client moved to a new area and felt disconnected, I suggested they ask for a Plant to help them connect with the Land. When a student identified a pattern they wanted to shift, I suggested they ask for a Plant to help. When I was looking for my home, I asked for a Plant to help me find ki. When my students begin their practices, they inevitably encounter client issues or patterns that I have not, and I remind them to ask for a Plant who can help. I have learned from incredible, generous humans, and there are endless possibilities in this world; no one person can give us all of the answers. The Plants, however, meet us exactly where we need them to. They can guide us through any issue. We simply need to ask and pay attention. Often, they show us what we need before we even know to ask for it.

Once we ask for a Plant to provide guidance, we become observant about who is "showing up." Look for a Plant who presents themselves three times or appears in strange ways. For instance, one of my students asked for a Plant. She visited her local conservatory during her lunch break and enjoyed their Orchid exhibit. On her walk back to work, she spotted an Orchid on the sidewalk (this was winter and no Orchids grew nearby). When she returned to work, there was leftover salad from a meeting. As she ate, she discovered an Orchid in her salad. Orchid was trying to get her attention. If a Plant appears three times, pay attention; ki has something to share. Sometimes it is clear before the third appearance. For example, as I drove to the bank today, a question came into my head, and I immediately saw a blooming Daisy. It is December in Pennsylvania, so this was extremely unusual. Daisy is the flower associated with a beloved client and student who died this year. Seeing this flower, I received the answer that I needed.

When you are comfortable communicating with Plants, you can communicate with the other Beings of Nature: rock, water, Forest, Faeries, or a particular Land. As we communicate, listen, and learn with our more-than-human relatives, we engage in co-creative partnership. We begin to create the world of our dreams together—a world where every action and every decision is based on Love, on the re-membering of our inherent connection to all. This work is what we are doing at Heart Springs Sanctuary.

Sometimes creating this world seems daunting. The changes that are needed seem immense. The systems feel too ingrained. We may not even be able to imagine this world, for ki seems like an impossibility. But this is all an illusion, for this world is already being formed. We may not see it on the news or in our government, but if you look, you can find ki among the incredible people choosing Love and dedicating their lives to living in co-creative partnership with Earth. We help to shape this world every time we communicate with Plants and our other relatives. Every time that we choose co-creative partnership, we give courage to others who want a shift. I am blessed to witness a growing number of people engaging in co-creative partnership with Nature. They give me hope that we will create a new story for humanity.

Love is the basis of my practice, my classes, and this book. When we choose Love, we change the vibration of this world. Sometimes these changes are small and sometimes they are large, touching many Hearts for generations (such as the work of Martin Luther King Jr.). The Plants will guide us on this path of Love, for that is the only way that humanity will thrive. The Plants help us to create a new story, a story based on Love and co-creative partnership. A story in which *all* Beings are honored and thrive. Together, we can rewrite our future and bring the world of our dreams into reality.

I asked the Plants for any final messages to share with you. They flashed through the many messages they have shared with me over the years, especially the ones that I have included in this book. They pointed out that every message, every lesson, and every moment is based in Love. We are always surrounded by Love. We are never alone. They said, "You are loved more than you will ever know." They ask that we allow our Hearts to open, to re-member our union with All, and choose Love. They say that in the darkest times, when all seems lost, turn to the Plants—they will be there.

And so, Dear Reader, thank you for joining me on this journey with the Plants. May you continue to re-member who you are. May you follow your Soul's path, allowing your Heart to lead the way. May this path be filled with beauty and grace. When it becomes challenging, may you remember that the Plants are there for support and guidance. Above all else, may you always know that you are Love(d).

❧ Acknowledgments ❧

*W*hen gratitude is the foundation for your work, it is a daunting task to write a concise acknowledgments section. My life and work have been influenced by so many, including complete strangers; I am grateful to everyone who has touched my Heart along the way.

My biggest gratitude, of course, must go to the Plants who not only provide my life, but have been incredible Guides and companions along the way and are the co-authors of this book. That gratitude circles out to the Nature Spirits, Faeries, and other Guides who support me every day and make this world astoundingly beautiful.

My life has been blessed by many human teachers and Guides who have encouraged me on my path, especially Rocío Alarcón, Don Babineau, David Dalton, Margi Flint, Kate Gilday, Rosemary Gladstar, and Tina Sams. Yes, their work has contributed to my own, but more than that their Beingness—who they are—touches my Heart and inspires me to be a better person. There are no words to express my overwhelming gratitude to my teacher, mentor, and dear friend Pam Montgomery for her incredible generosity and encouragement, including some much-needed kicks in the butt. Quite frankly, Pam saved my life. She has shown me what it means to stand in Integrity and dedicate your life to Earth. One of my greatest honors is working with her to create a better future for All, including through our work with the Organization of Nature Evolutionaries (O.N.E).

I thank the many hands and eyes that helped to bring this book into fruition including the beautiful people at Inner Traditions • Bear & Company: Erica Robinson, Manzanita Carpenter Sanz, Sharon Reed, and especially Jon Graham for giving me the encouragement to share the Plants' messages and Lyz Perry for her guidance, patience, and wisdom which enhanced this book. Gratitude to Lisa Brinton for being an early reader and editor. I also thank my lifelong proofreader and mother, Mary Dissinger, whose Love, support, and courage helped to form me and gave me the confidence to be me. I have enormous gratitude for Susan Boyd, who has been on this journey with me for many years, never letting me forget that there is a book that needs to be written. Susan's dedication and wisdom buoyed me when I was floundering. Without a doubt, she improved this book and helped me to be a better writer. Deep gratitude goes as well to the amazingly talented Lillian Edwards, who translated my words into gorgeous illustrations that are truly Love letters honoring the Plants. I greatly appreciate her intuition and deep devotion; it is a blessing to walk this path with her. You can learn more about her work at www.earthprayer.love.

To my clients and students, I thank you for your trust and dedication. You allow me to continue this work with the Plants and have taught me much over these years. It is an honor to witness you in your Becoming.

Much gratitude goes to my motley crew of a family, especially my grandparents, who taught me about Love and invited me into the magical world of Plants, and to my children, who are possibly my biggest teachers, propelling me to do my personal work. Through them, I learned that there is no limit to Love. Gratitude also goes to my two fathers: my biological father, Bernie, and my father of the Heart (step-father), Barry. They are both mentioned in the book, though I did not distinguish them. They have very different personalities and roles in my life and I am truly blessed to be surrounded by their Love and support. Thank you also to my lifelong cheerleaders, my Aunts Dawn and Dianne.

I also send great gratitude to my spiritual family, especially my incredible si-Stars Barbara, Jen, Jody, Kim, Lisa, Marjorie, and Tonya who have picked me up off the floor, never let me forget my crown, and pushed me when needed. The full list of my si-Stars is too long to name. I thank each of you who helped me create a beautiful life beyond my dreams. You have been by my side through some of the most difficult times, never let me dim my light, reminded me to dance and laugh, fed me good food, and taught me how to be in a community that uplifts one another. May everyone be blessed with friends like you.

I am forever grateful for the beautiful gift of my partner, Marcus Sheffer. There are many, many hours that go into writing a book. Marcus has fed me, encouraged me, and supported me through them all including taking care of everything else so that I could focus on writing. He has read and re-read, inspired me, helped me process my thoughts, and been completely steadfast throughout this process. I truly have never felt more loved and am grateful for his presence in my life.

Finally, I thank you, Dear Reader, and everyone who is answering the call of the Plants and of Nature to return to the family and create the Garden of our re-membering. You give me hope. Together we thrive. May our Hearts be One.

❧ Notes ☙

Introduction: An Invitation into the Plant World

1. Kimmerer, "Nature Needs a New Pronoun."

1. Plant Communication

1. Childre and Howard, *The HeartMath Solution,* 19.

2. Taste the Wild: Mulberry

1. Van der Kolk, "Trauma, the Body, and 2021."

3. New Opportunity: Yarrow

1. Roads, *Through the Eyes of Love: Book One,* 156.
2. hooks, *The Will to Change,* 66.

4. Dare to Dream: Mugwort

1. Montgomery, *Plant Spirit Healing,* 181.
2. United Plant Savers, "Species At-Risk List."
3. Mountain Dreamer, "The Invitation," 1.
4. Moss, *Dreaming the Soul Back Home,* 117.

5. Becoming the Authority: Plantain

1. Penniman, *Farming While Black,* 309.
2. Center for Nonviolent Communication, "Feelings Inventory."

6. Resiliency: Dandelion

1. Gandhi, *The Gift of Anger,* 18.
2. Sales, "Where Does It Hurt?"
3. DiFranco, "Buildings and Bridges."

7. Sweetness of Life: Maple

1. Kimmerer, *Braiding Sweetgrass,* 111.
2. Movement Generation, "From Banks and Tanks," 4.

10. Changing Our Story: Black-Eyed Susan

1. Van der Kolk, *The Body Keeps the Score,* 193.
2. Lipton, *The Biology of Belief,* 98.
3. Menakem, "Notice the Rage; Notice the Silence."
4. Van der Kolk, *The Body Keeps the Score,* 21.
5. Walker, *Complex PTSD,* 332–34.
6. Van der Kolk, *The Body Keeps the Score,* 150.
7. Van der Kolk, *The Body Keeps the Score,* 56.
8. Korotkov, "Prof. Fritz-Albert Popp."
9. Chang and Popp, "Biological Organization," 217.

11. Releasing Grief: Willow

1. Montgomery, *Plant Spirit Healing,* 103.
2. Montgomery, *Partner Earth,* 132.
3. Prechtel, *The Smell of Rain on Dust,* 75.

12. Power of Love: Rose

1. Strand and Finn, *The Way of the Rose,* 80.

2. Strand and Finn, *The Way of the Rose*, 81.
3. Roads, *Through the Eyes of Love: Book Three*, 126.
4. Peck, *The Road Less Traveled*, 81.
5. hooks, *All About Love*, 6.
6. Taylor, *The Body Is Not an Apology*, 7.

13. Living to Die: Poison Hemlock

1. Roads, *Through the Eyes of Love: Book One*, 212–13.
2. Walker, *Complex PTSD*, 7–8.
3. *Encyclopædia Britannica*, "Shamanism."

14. Everything Changes: Eastern Hemlock

1. Aluli Meyer, "Ku'u 'Aina Aloha, My Beloved Land," 93.
2. Lipton and Bhaerman, *Spontaneous Evolution*, 121–12.
3. Bach. *The Essential Writings of Dr. Edward Bach*, 4.

15. The Great Mother: Corn

1. Lancaster County Agricultural Council, "Conservation."
2. Pollan, *The Omnivores' Dilemma*, 24–25.
3. Penniman, *Farming While Black*, 152.
4. Prechtel, *The Unlikely Peace at Cuchumaquic*, Dedication.
5. Shiva, "Introduction," 1.
6. Prechtel, *The Unlikely Peace at Cuchumaquic*, 155.
7. Gardening Channel, "Corn vs. Maize."
8. Williams, *When Women Were Birds*, 225.

16. Re-membering a New Way: Rosemary

1. Childre and Howard, *The HeartMath Solution*, 125.
2. Goleman, *Social Intelligence*, 288.
3. Ruiz, *The Four Agreements*, 47.
4. Goldman, *Gift of the Body*, 313.
5. Van der Kolk, "Trauma, the Body, and 2021."

6. Montgomery, *Plant Spirit Healing,* 174.

7. Montgomery, *Plant Spirit Healing,* 172.

8. Soulé, "The Social Siege of Nature," 141–42.

17. Becoming Sacred Humans: Tulsi

1. Rai, *Holy Basil,* 11.

2. Rai, *Holy Basil,* 15.

3. Bly, *A Little Book on the Human Shadow,* 18.

4. Montgomery, *Plant Spirit Healing,* 52.

5. Tello, *Recovering Your Sacredness,* 151.

6. Guyett, *Sacred Plant Initiations,* 2.

7. Guyett, *Sacred Plant Initiations,* 21.

Bibliography

Aluli Meyer, Manulani. "Ku'u 'Aina Aloha, My Beloved Land: Interspecies Kinship in Hawai'i." In *Kinship: Belonging In a World of Relations Vol. 01 Planet*, edited by Gavin Van Horn, Robin Wall Kimmerer, and John Hausdoerffer, 84–100. Libertyville, Ill.: Center for Humans and Nature Press, 2021.

Bach, Edward. *The Essential Writings of Dr Edward Bach: The Twelve Healers and Heal Thyself.* London: Vermilion, 2005.

Bioneers website. "Eve Ensler: The Alchemy of the Apology." Accessed November 19, 2022.

Bly, Robert. *A Little Book on the Human Shadow.* Edited by William Booth. New York: Harper One, 1988.

Center for Nonviolent Communication website. "Feelings Inventory." Accessed December 31, 2021.

Chang, Jiin-Ju, and Fritz-Albert Popp. "Biological Organization: A Possible Mechanism Based on the Coherence of 'Biophotons.'" In *Biophotons*, edited by Jiin-Ju Chang, Joachim Fisch, and Fritz-Albert Popp, 217–27. Dordrecht, Netherlands: Springer Dordrecht, 1988.

Childre, Doc, and Howard Martin with Donna Beech. *The HeartMath Solution.* New York: Harper Collins, 1999.

Dalton, David. *Stars of the Meadow: Medicinal Herbs as Flower Essences.* Great Barrington, Mass.: Lindisfarne Books, 2006.

DiFranco, Ani. "Buildings and Bridges." Track 1 on *Out of Range.* Righteous Babe Records, 1994, CD.

Encyclopædia Britannica website. "Shamanism." Accessed October 21, 2021.

Gandhi, Arun. *The Gift of Anger.* New York: Gallery Books/Jeter Publishing, 2017.

Gardening Channel website. "Corn vs. Maize, What's the Difference?" Accessed November 2, 2020.

Geniusz, Mary Siisip. *Plants Have So Much to Give Us, All We Have to Do Is Ask: Anishinaabe Botanical Teachings.* Minneapolis: University of Minnesota Press, 2015.

Goldman, Jonathan M. *Gift of the Body: A Multi-Dimensional Guide to Energy Anatomy, Grounded Spirituality and Living Through the Heart.* Bend, Ore.: Essential Light Institute, 2014.

Goleman, Daniel. *Social Intelligence: The Revolutionary New Science of Human Relationships.* New York: Bantam Books, 2007.

Guyett, Carole. *Sacred Plant Initiations: Communicating with Plants for Healing and Higher Consciousness.* Rochester, Vt.: Bear & Company, 2015.

Holmes, Peter. *The Energetics of Western Herbs.* Cotati, Calif.: Snow Lotus Press, 2007.

hooks, bell. *All About Love: New Visions.* New York: William Morrow, 2001.

———. *The Will to Change: Men, Masculinity, and Love.* New York: Washington Square Press, 2004.

Kimmerer, Robin Wall. *Braiding Sweetgrass: Indigenous Wisdom, Scientific Knowledge, and the Teachings of Plants.* Minneapolis, Minn.: Milkweed Editions, 2013.

———. "Nature Needs a New Pronoun: To Stop the Age of Extinction, Let's Start by Ditching 'It.'" *YES! Magazine,* March 30, 2015.

Korotkov, Konstantin. "Prof. Fritz-Albert Popp – IUMAB Father of the Biophotonics." IUMAB. August 10, 2018.

Lancaster County Agriculture Council website. "Conservation." Last modified March 15, 2021.

Lee, Michele E. *Working the Roots: Over 400 Years of Traditional African-American Healing.* Oakland, Calif.: Wadastick Publishers, 2014.

Lipton, Bruce H. *The Biology of Belief: Unleashing the Power of Consciousness, Matter, & Miracles.* New York City: Hay House, 2012.

Lipton, Bruce H. and Steven Bhaerman. *Spontaneous Evolution: Our Positive Future (And a Way to Get There from Here).* Carlsbad, Calif.: Hay House, 2009.

McIntyre, Anne. *Flower Power.* New York: Henry Holt and Company, 1996.

Menakem, Resmaa. "Notice the Rage; Notice the Silence." Interview with Krista Tippett. The On Being Project, June 4, 2020.

Moerman, Daniel E. *Native American Medicinal Plants*. Portland, Ore.: Timber Press, 2009.

Montgomery, Pam. *Partner Earth: A Spiritual Ecology*. Rochester, Vt.: Destiny Books, 1997.

———. *Plant Spirit Healing: A Guide to Working with Plant Consciousness*. Rochester, Vt.: Bear & Company, 2008.

Moss, Robert. *Dreaming the Soul Back Home: Shamanic Dreaming for Healing and Becoming Whole*. Novato, Calif.: New World Library, 2012.

Mountain Dreamer, Oriah. "The Invitation." In *The Invitation* by Oriah Mountain Dreamer, 1–2. San Francisco: HarperSanFrancisco, 1999.

Movement Generation Justice and Ecology Project. "From Banks and Tanks to Cooperation and Caring: A Strategic Framework for a Just Transition." Zine. 2016.

Peck, M. Scott. *The Road Less Traveled: A New Psychology of Love, Traditional Values, and Spiritual Growth*. New York: Simon and Schuster, 1978.

Penniman, Leah. *Farming While Black: Soul Fire Farm's Practical Guide to Liberation on the Land*. White River Junction, Vt.: Chelsea Green Publishing, 2018.

Pollan, Michael. *The Omnivore's Dilemma: A Natural History of Four Meals*. New York: Penguin Books, 2006.

Prechtel, Martín. *The Smell of Rain on Dust: Grief and Praise*. Berkeley, Calif.: North Atlantic Books, 2015.

———. *The Unlikely Peace at Cuchumaquic: The Parallel Lives of People as Plants: Keeping the Seeds Alive*. Berkeley, Calif.: North Atlantic Books, 2012.

Rai, Yash. *Holy Basil: Tulsi (A Herb)*. Ahmadabad, India: Navneet Publications (India) Limited, 2007.

Roads, Michael J. *Through the Eyes of Love: Journeying with Pan, Book One*. 2nd ed. Portland, Ore.: Six Degrees Publishing Group, 2013.

———. *Through the Eyes of Love: Journeying with Pan, Book Three*. Portland, Ore: Six Degrees Publishing Group, 2012.

Ruiz, Don Miguel. *The Four Agreements: A Practical Guide to Personal Freedom*. San Rafael, Calif.: Amber-Allen Publishing, 1997.

Sales, Ruby. "Where Does It Hurt?" Interview with Krista Tippett. The On Being Project, June 2, 2020.

Shiva, Vandana. "Introduction." In *Sacred Seed*, 1–6, Point Reyes, Calif.: The Golden Sufi Center Publishing, 2014.

Soulé, Michael. "Social Siege of Nature." In *Reinventing Nature? Responses to Postmodern Deconstruction,* edited by Michael Soulé and Gary Lease, 136–70. San Francisco: Island Press, 1995.

Strand, Clark, and Perdita Finn. *The Way of the Rose: The Radical Path of the Divine Feminine Hidden in the Rosary.* New York: Random House, 2019.

Taylor, Sonya Renee. *The Body Is Not an Apology: The Power of Radical Self-Love, Second Edition.* Oakland, Calif.: Berrett-Koehler Publishers, 2021.

Tello, Jerry. *Recovering Your Sacredness: Ancestral Teachings for Today's Living.* Hacienda Heights, Calif.: Sueños Publications, 2018.

United Plant Savers. "Species At-Risk List." Last modified February 20, 2021.

Van der Kolk, Bessel. *The Body Keeps the Score: Brain, Mind, and Body in the Healing of Trauma.* New York: Penguin Books, 2014.

———. "Trauma, the Body, and 2021." Interview with Krista Tippett. The On Being Project, November 11, 2021.

Walker, Pete. *Complex PTSD: From Surviving to Thriving.* Lafayette, Calif.: Azure Coyote Publishing, 2013.

Watterson, Kathryn. *Not by the Sword: How a Cantor and His Family Transformed a Klansman.* University of Nebraska Press, Bison Books, 2012.

Williams, Terry Tempest. *When Women Were Birds: Fifty-four Variations on Voice.* New York: Picador, 2012.

Wood, Matthew. *The Book of Herbal Wisdom.* Berkeley, Calif.: North Atlantic Books, 1997.

∞ Index ∞

Books of Related Interest

Plant Spirit Healing
A Guide to Working with Plant Consciousness
by Pam Montgomery

Sacred Plant Initiations
Communicating with Plants for Healing and Higher Consciousness
by Carole Guyett
Foreword by Pam Montgomery

Journeys with Plant Spirits
Plant Consciousness Healing and Natural Magic Practices
by Emma Farrell
Foreword by Pam Montgomery

The Secret Teachings of Plants
The Intelligence of the Heart in the Direct Perception of Nature
by Stephen Harrod Buhner

Plant Intelligence and the Imaginal Realm
Beyond the Doors of Perception into the Dreaming of Earth
by Stephen Harrod Buhner

Plant Spirit Reiki
Energy Healing with the Elements of Nature
by Fay Johnstone

Encounters with Nature Spirits
Co-creating with the Elemental Kingdom
by R. Ogilvie Crombie

Secret Medicines from Your Garden
Plants for Healing, Spirituality, and Magic
by Ellen Evert Hopman

INNER TRADITIONS • BEAR & COMPANY
P.O. Box 388
Rochester, VT 05767
1-800-246-8648
www.InnerTraditions.com

Or contact your local bookseller